P9-DXN-401

THE ZONE

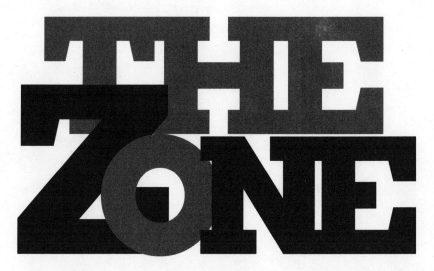

A Dietary Road Map

Barry Sears, Ph.D.

with Bill Lawren

ReganBooks
An Imprint of HarperCollinsPublishers

THE ZONE. Copyright © 1995 by Barry Sears and William Lawren. All rights reserved. Printed in the United States of America. No part of this book may be used or reproduced in any manner whatsoever without written permission except in the case of brief quotations embodied in critical articles and reviews. For more information address HarperCollins Publishers, Inc. 10 East 53rd Street, New York, NY 10022.

HarperCollins books may be purchased for educational, business, or sales promotional use. For information please write: Special Markets Department, HarperCollins Publishers, Inc., 10 East 53rd Street, New York, NY 10022.

FIRST EDITION

Designed by Nancy Singer

Library of Congress Cataloging-in-Publication Data

Sears, Barry. 1947–
    The zone : a revolutionary life plan to put your body in total balance for permanent weight loss / Barry Sears, with Bill Lawren—1st ed.
        p.   cm.
    ISBN 0-06-039150-2
    1. Reducing   2. Nutrition.   I. Lawren, Bill.   II. Title.
RM222.2.S39   1995
613.2′5—dc20   95-17096

98 99   CC/RRD   80 79 78

CONTENTS

ACKNOWLEDGMENTS

No one works in isolation, and the twelve-year journey that led to this book attests to that fact. I want to thank my family, beginning with my wife, Lynn Sears. She not only helped tremendously on the editing of the book, but also believed in me twelve years ago when I told her that I was leaving MIT to work on "something really big." Her support and perseverance have been godsends.

Likewise, I am indebted to my brother, Doug, my partner, confidant, and, next to my wife, my closest friend, even after I enticed him to leave a promising career in the computer industry to work with me on "something really big." During those two bleak winters in Saskatoon, as we learned to grow and process borage seeds, I am sure he had second thoughts.

I must also thank my very first employee, my mother, who has been an integral stabilizing influence in every one of my business enterprises since we started in 1976.

There are the various other individuals who not only shared my vision but provided the commitment without which none of this work would have been completed. These include Harry Haveles, John Mouganis and Mike Palm. Likewise, physicians like Paul Kahl, Sam Golden, Michael and Mary Dan Eades, Michael Norden and Daniel Wistran—they had the courage to believe in new approaches for the treatment and prevention of disease.

There are also the coaches: Garrett Giemont, Marv Marinovich, Skip Kenney, and Richard Quick. They took big chances with their athletes on this dietary technology because of their conviction that this technology could extend the limits of human performance. I must also thank all the individuals I have worked with over the years. Their feedback has been instrumental in refining my technology to its current state.

Finally, I am grateful for the support and vision of Judith Regan, who brought my research to the general public, and to Dr. Jeffrey Schwartz, who initially introduced my technology to Judith.

PREFACE

A sword of Damocles hangs over my head, something I've known since my early twenties. You see, I'm a walking genetic time bomb. I'm genetically programmed by nature to die of heart disease within the next ten years. My early death seems all but inevitable: my grandfather, father, and every one of my three uncles were killed by heart attacks before they reached the age of fifty-four.

As I write this, I'm forty-seven.

The genes that are killing the men in my family are insidious. To look at us, no one could imagine that we are—or were—anything but healthy and hearty. My father, Dale Sears, was a great athlete in the 1940s. At only six feet two inches tall, he was an All-American basketball center at the University of Southern California, as he liked to say, "the last of the six-foot centers." He was chosen to play on the U.S. Olympic basketball team in 1940, but World War II robbed him of his Olympic opportunity. (I myself played college basketball, and continued playing volleyball at the national level for some time after receiving my Ph.D.)

After the war, my dad went into the floor-covering business with one of my uncles. He gained about twenty pounds and he smoked, but he was still active and in reasonably good shape. He continued to play basketball, and took up volleyball on the side.

When he was just forty-three, he had his first heart attack. I was thirteen at the time, and all I remember is that he spent a few days in the hospital. The doctors said it was a relatively mild attack, and he recuperated at home for another six weeks. Like all teen-agers, I wasn't much inclined to worry about health problems, even my father's. And he didn't seem too concerned either.

The next ten years brought more danger signs: two of my uncles had heart attacks. Then, when he was only fifty-three, my father had a second, fatal attack. There was no warning. He died in his sleep. During the next few years, my three uncles all died of heart attacks. They were all in their early fifties.

By then I could hear a clear message. If I didn't do something, I'd become an early victim too. So I did the normal things: tried to stay in shape by maintaining a highly athletic lifestyle, kept my weight under control, and ate what I thought was a healthy diet. But with my unfortunate genetics, I suspected that even that would not be enough.

I realized that to save my own life I would have to know much more. I needed to know what made the difference between a healthy heart and a heart so genetically flawed it would only last two-thirds of a normal lifetime.

By then I had already earned a Ph.D. in biochemistry from Indiana University. I was doing postdoctoral work at the University of Virginia, looking at the molecular structure of lipids, the medical name for the class of compounds that includes, among others, cholesterol and the so-called lipoproteins: HDL, LDL, and VLDL.

Up to then, my research had been pure basic science. I wanted to see how these complex molecules were put together. But my father's death (and my own sense of impending doom) shifted my direction. Instead of just looking at the molecular architecture of cholesterol and its relatives, I decided to look at their role in heart disease. It was the early 1970s and, scientifically speaking, the study of cholesterol and its relationship to heart trouble was just getting off the ground. Still, it was already a hot and emerging medical field.

I knew a lot about lipids, but virtually nothing about heart disease. So I moved on to Boston University School of Medicine to work with Don Small, who was performing ground-breaking research on how the structure of lipids might be contributing to cardiovascular disease. I ensconced myself in the university medical library, reading anything I could find on the subject. I had no preconceptions, no base of knowledge to work from, so I read everything.

I eventually came across an obscure report. At San Francisco's Mount Zion Hospital, two researchers, Sanford Byers and Meyer Friedman, had induced atherosclerosis—the clogging and hardening of the arteries that often leads to heart attacks—in rabbits by feeding the animals a diet high in saturated fat. Then half the animals were injected with the same phospholipids I had studied for my Ph.D. dissertation. The results were astonishing. The phospholipid injections acted like a biological Roto-Rooter, completely clearing most of the animals' clogged arteries, in effect erasing all traces of heart disease.

My interest was already starting to be rewarded. But this report appeared in a very obscure journal, so I continued reading. Soon I found an equally obscure report in which Jonas Maurukas and Robert Thomas had replicated the earlier work with phospholipids—not to see if it was right, but to prove it wrong. (In fact, almost all the noted researchers seemed to think the earlier work was idiotic. How could you eliminate heart disease simply by injecting phospholipids into animals?) These investigators were going to use a better animal model and better techniques to prove how wrong this early report was. Much to their surprise, they got the same results—elimination of all traces of atherosclerotic lesions.

Similar results continued to appear in scientific literature about every three to five years. Then in 1975 researchers at Upjohn published definitive research confirming these isolated reports. In essence, heart disease could be reduced, if not eradicated, through a simple injection of the natural lipids that are the basis of every cell in the body. This was real biotechnology! Since I was one of the few scientists studying phospholipids at that time, I thought I was going to go to the head of the class—not to mention save my own life.

When the Upjohn scientists published their research, it should have been big news. It should have touched off a furious race among the giant drug companies to develop and market phospholipids as a treatment for heart disease in humans. But it didn't. The drug manufacturers had a business problem: phospholipids are natural substances, and it's impossible to get a patent for something that occurs in nature. Without the possibility of the exclusive rights a patent confers, the drug companies, including Upjohn, were not interested.

But I was. Younger and more naïve then, I thought the only thing I needed to cure atherosclerosis was to develop a patentable phospholipid. This newly created substance would act like a chemical Roto-Rooter (just like a natural phospholipid), sucking the cholesterol from artery-clogging plaques and carrying it to the liver, where it would be metabolized like garbage in an incinerator. If I could turn this trick, I realized, it might not only save my own life, it could also help lengthen the lives of millions of heart-disease patients. And, of course, in the process I would become a pharmaceutical tycoon.

As I would soon discover, life is never quite that easy or straightforward.

Through my research background, I already knew quite a bit about how to change the molecular structure of phospholipids. Making small changes in that structure, I could produce a phospholipid-like substance that could be patented. That, I thought, should prove interesting to the big drug companies, which had the money and the facilities to take a phospholipid drug to the public. I went to my funding partners—my mother, my father-in-law, and my aunts and uncles—and in 1976 started one of the first biotech companies: Lipid Specialties, Inc. I rented lab space in downtown Boston and started working with a single technician to eradicate heart disease.

By tweaking the phospholipid molecule—adding a carbon atom here, a methyl group there—I soon created a series of "new" phospholipids. These molecules were at least slightly unlike anything seen in nature, and therefore patentable.

Sure that I was on the brink of a cure for heart disease, I patented the new molecules and took them to Upjohn. The drug-company researchers tested these phospholipids on the same atherosclerotic Japanese quails that they had used in their own studies. My phospholipids had virtually the same effect as the natural variety: they reduced the amount of plaque on the animals' artery walls.

But a slight complication was occurring—some of the animals were dying. It turned out that the patentable phospholipids I had made were too good. They were pulling cholesterol from the atherosclerotic lesions, but they were also pulling the cholesterol from the red blood cells. These cells then ruptured and leaked hemoglobin—the substance that carries oxygen to the cells. This was killing some of the animals. Once I saw the results, I knew immediately how to solve the problem. Only two things stood in my way. One was that I had run out of money, the second was Upjohn.

Upjohn wasn't interested in any further work. Why? Because our new phospholipids had to be injected in order to remove the cholesterol from the atherosclerotic lesion, and Upjohn's upper management didn't want to deal with any potential cardiovascular drug that couldn't be made into a pill.

So much for my dreams of being financially solvent, let alone a pharmaceutical tycoon. And, of course, my own biological time bomb was still ticking.

Still, I had learned a valuable lesson: when it comes to treating heart disease, think of something you can swallow or eat.

All was not lost. I still had all this new and patentable phospholipid technology. What I needed was a partner. As luck would have it, I came across my mentor in drug-delivery technology, David Yesair. David was a vice president at Arthur D. Little, a major consulting company in Boston. He was uninterested in heart disease, but was passionate about cancer treatment.

David's cancer-fighting drugs at the time were great antitumor agents in the test tube, but because they were so water-insoluble, they could never be injected into humans. No problem: I now had a patentable technology to solve this dilemma. So rather than sucking cholesterol from atherosclerotic lesions, I used this phospholipid technology to deliver new and unusual anticancer drugs with greater specificity and less toxicity than ever before imagined. (One of these drugs, by the way, was AZT, now among the only drugs approved to treat people with AIDS.)

Since that time, I have continued to evolve my drug-delivery technology to solve many of the inherent problems associated with cancer drugs (I now hold most of the major patents in the world for intravenous cancer-drug delivery).

But all this still did nothing for my heart, which was not getting any younger. To make things worse, in 1984 I had a personal wake-up call: I was hospitalized for a week with cardiac arrhythmias. Needless to say, my interest in treating heart disease was intensifying.

But I could see the light at the end of the tunnel. In 1982 news came from Oslo that would change both the direction of my research and the course of my life. That year's Nobel Prize for Physiology and Medicine was awarded to Sune Bergstrom and Bengt Samuelsson of the Karolinska Institute in Stockholm and John Vane of the Royal College of Surgeons in England for research on the powerful class of hormones called *eicosanoids*. (Remember this word. You'll hear it again and again in the course of this book. It's pronounced eye-KAH-sah-noids.) Actually, Vane's part of the Nobel Prize was based on his research on aspirin—that's right, plain old garden-variety aspirin.

At the time, virtually no one outside the world of lipid research (and that's a very small world) had ever heard of their work. Before the three prize-winning scientists came along, everyone knew at least some of the things that aspirin does—it reduces pain, controls fever, etc.—but no one really knew how it works its magic in the body. Bergstrom, Samuelsson, and Vane's award-winning work solved the mystery: aspirin works its wonders by affecting eicosanoids.

These hormones—there are hundreds of them—are among the most powerful and important substances in the body. They act as "master switches" that control virtually all human body functions—including the cardiovascular system, the immune system, and the systems that govern how much fat we store (and therefore how much we weigh). Eicosanoids are so crucial to our health and well-being that I came to think of them as the "molecular glue" that holds the human body together.

I first became aware of eicosanoids during my research on lipids. Certain fatty acids associated with natural lipids are also the building blocks of eicosanoids. But Bergstrom, Samuelsson, and Vane's Nobel Prize–winning research opened my eyes to how important eicosanoids really are. It occurred to me that if someone could control eicosanoids, they would actually control virtually every aspect of human physiology, including the cardiovascular system.

It also occurred to me that since eicosanoids are involved in virtually everything the body does, controlling them might represent a new paradigm for health and illness. It seemed to make sense that many of our disease states—heart disease, diabetes, arthritis, and cancer, to name just a few—might be the result of imbalances among the eicosanoid hormones.

If that were true, restoring and maintaining a proper balance of eicosanoids might help prevent or even become the primary treatment for these diseases. Even better, it might help maintain a state of nearly perpetual good health: a molecular definition of "wellness" that would lead to a better quality of life. As an ultimate payoff, keeping eicosanoids in balance might help all of us reach that near-euphoric state of maximum physical, mental, and psychological performance that athletes call "the Zone."

Now everyone knows that in the athletic context the Zone is a fleeting thing—it's extremely hard to reach. Even when an athlete gets there, it rarely lasts longer than a few minutes. (I found it myself a few times when I played at the national volleyball championships, but my time in the Zone was usually measured in seconds.) The key to reaching the Zone and staying in it, I realized, might lie in controlling the balance of eicosanoid hormones. I began to wonder if it might even be possible to stretch the duration of the Zone—to reach it whenever we wanted and then to *stay* in it, not just for a few minutes (or a few games), but twenty-four hours a day for the rest of our lives.

In cancer-drug delivery there is a Zone too, known as the therapeutic zone. When a concentration of cancer drug is too low, it is ineffective. If the concentration is too high, it is toxic. At the right level, it is therapeutic. Like the Zone in athletics, the therapeutic zone for a cancer drug can be exceedingly narrow. So I figured that this eicosanoid Zone I was searching for would probably combine properties of the Zone taken from both the athletic context (optimum performance) and the context of cancer-drug delivery (defined mathematical limits).

The question, of course, was how to accomplish all this? I knew that eicosanoids couldn't just be injected into the bloodstream like cancer drugs. They're so powerful they would simply overwhelm the body, throwing all its important physiological systems dangerously haywire. This is why major drug companies like Upjohn, Burroughs Wellcome, and Ono had spent billions of dollars on eicosanoid research but had no drugs to show for it.

I decided to approach eicosanoids from a different perspective— at the level of the individual cell, where the eicosanoids are manufactured in the first place. My goal was to learn how to tip the balance of the molecular building blocks of eicosanoids in the cell membranes so that the cells would manufacture the right types of eicosanoids to reach the Zone.

How could I do this? By applying the drug-delivery principles I was already using for cancer drugs to the ideal oral drug-delivery system for eicosanoids: food. That's it in a nutshell, and that's what this book is all about—using food to manipulate eicosanoid balance, and using that balance as a passport to the Zone. In the following chapters I'll explain in detail how I learned to break this nutritional code, and how I've continued to refine it until it's now finally ready for public consumption.

How do I know it's ready? Because I've now spent almost six years developing this dietary program, testing it on the only species that counts: human beings. From my first human "guinea pigs" (myself, my brother, Doug, and my wife), I've gone on to test and refine this eicosanoid-favorable nutritional system on world-class athletes—including the Stanford University swim teams, elite triathletes, and various NFL, NBA, and professional baseball players. I've also tested it on people with some of our nastiest killer diseases, including diabetes, heart disease, and AIDS. In addition, the program has been tried by hundreds of ordinary people who simply wanted to lose weight and feel their best.

My results have convinced me that this dietary technology is the most powerful means ever discovered to help people achieve that state of optimal good health, physical performance, and mental alertness that's called the Zone.

I'm now convinced that reaching the Zone and staying in it can help prevent heart disease. It should even help reverse heart disease when it does occur. Staying in the Zone is your best defense to ward off cancer, and has a positive impact on a host of other diseases, including diabetes, arthritis, "mental" diseases like depression and alcoholism, even chronic fatigue.

In fact, reaching the Zone and maintaining it should ultimately help us reach that most universal of personal goals: to live longer, healthier, and more satisfying lives. In the bargain, staying in the Zone will keep us performing at our absolute best—hour after hour, day after day, month after month—for the rest of our lives.

These are not unique claims. The proponents of every new diet that comes along say essentially the same thing. But if you're reading this book, you probably already know that these diets don't really work. You may have already tried one of today's trendy, low-fat, low-protein, high-carbohydrate diets and been disappointed with the results. Well, the fact is that for a number of reasons these diets can't possibly work. They can't help you lose weight in a permanent way, and they can't boost your physical performance—even if that's exactly what they're designed to do.

In fact, I'm now firmly convinced that these high-carb diets can actually be dangerous, that they can actually help bring on the diseases they're supposed to prevent. Why? Because they violate the basic biochemical laws required to enter the Zone.

The beauty of the dietary system presented in this book is that it's doable. It doesn't require that you eat anything weird, and it doesn't call for a great deal of the kind of unrealistic self-sacrifice that causes many people to fall off the diet wagon. It doesn't rob food of most of its flavor, as do many of the extremely low-fat diets. In fact, I can even show you how to stay within these dietary guidelines while eating at fast-food restaurants. And yes, you can still have your Häagen-Dazs.

Think of this book as having two distinct parts. The first portion gives you the rules and dietary tools to reach the Zone. The second part goes into greater detail on the health-care implications for living in the Zone, specifically with regard to chronic disease states such as heart disease, cancer, and others.

I hope this book serves as a wake-up call for both health-care professionals and the general public. I hope it will help reverse the growing health-care disaster stemming from the high-carbohydrate diets now being pushed on the American public.

Understanding the implications of the Zone can completely change your life. All you have to do is read this book, follow the simple dietary guidelines it recommends, and put them to work for you in your own life.

You'll be glad you did.

This book is not intended to replace medical advice or be a substitute for a physician. If you are sick or suspect you are sick, you should see a physician. If you are taking a prescription medication, you should never change your diet (for better or worse) without consulting your physician as any dietary change will affect the metabolism of that prescription drug. As powerful as modern medicine is, it remains a poor substitute for prevention.

Prevention will always be the best medicine. However, prevention can only be undertaken by the individual and that includes eating correctly. This is the foundation of a healthy lifestyle. You have to eat, so you might as well eat wisely.

Although this book is about food, the Authors and the Publisher expressly disclaim responsibility for any adverse effects arising from the use of nutritional supplements to your diet without appropriate medical supervision.

CHAPTER ONE

LIFE IN THE ZONE

Have you ever had one of those days when everything goes right? You wake up feeling alert, refreshed, and full of energy. You go off to work, finding open spaces that allow you to cruise through the rush-hour traffic. At your desk or out in the field, the solution to a problem that just yesterday seemed insoluble suddenly presents itself, seemingly out of thin air.

One by one, the tasks of the day surrender to your clear, efficient, yet apparently effortless approach. At your late-afternoon racquetball game (or jog, or aerobic workout) you're light on your feet and tireless. When you get home the kids are glad to see you—even your teenage son, the one with the ring in his nose—and when they get into one of their inevitable fights, you're there to adjudicate with the calm and wisdom of Solomon. After dinner, instead of collapsing in front of the TV, you have so much leftover energy that you're ready to go dancing.

You may not have put it to yourself this way, but you were probably in the Zone—that mysterious but very real state in which your body and mind work together at their ultimate best. Normally, we hear about the Zone in the context of athletics: a baseball player swears he can count the seams on a 90-mph fastball; a basketball player sees the hoop as twice its real size; a gymnast feels as if the balance beam is as wide as a city street.

In the Zone, the mind is relaxed, yet alert and exquisitely focused. Meanwhile, the body is fluid, strong, and apparently indefatigable. It's almost euphoric. There are no distractions, and time seems to slow down to a graceful waltz.

The legendary soccer player Pelé may have described the Zone best: "I felt a strange calmness," he wrote in his book *My Life and the Beautiful Game*, ". . . a kind of euphoria. I felt I could run all day without tiring, that I could dribble through any of their team or all of them, that I could almost pass through them physically. I felt I could

1

not be hurt. It was a very strange feeling and one I had not felt before. Perhaps it was merely confidence, but I have felt confident many times without that strange feeling of invincibility."

Most athletes—even those of us who are mere weekend warriors—have experienced this almost transcendent state at least once, and the experience is unforgettable. But there's nothing mystical about the Zone. *The Zone is a real metabolic state that can be reached by everyone, and maintained indefinitely on a lifelong basis.*

What is the Zone? Simply put, it's the metabolic state in which the body works at peak efficiency. Outside the Zone, life is its normal self—sometimes rewarding, mostly frustrating, filled with perplexing problems, missed opportunities, and illnesses great and small. But inside the Zone life becomes easier and better. In the Zone you'll enjoy optimal body function: freedom from hunger, greater energy and physical performance, as well as improved mental focus and productivity.

In the Zone, problems don't go away, but their solutions become more obvious. Fatigue and listlessness are replaced by feelings of energy and high competence. Weight loss (which should really be called fat loss) can be an ongoing and usually frustrating struggle for most people. In the Zone it is painless, almost automatic.

Life in the Zone creates significant health benefits. The little illnesses that plague us all—colds, flus, allergies—seem to happen less often. When they do hit, they're not as severe. And some of our more serious chronic diseases—heart disease and cancer, for example—become less likely to strike. And if these diseases do occur, in the Zone their treatment is more manageable.

In fact, being in the Zone can become the basis for a new kind of low-cost yet ultra-effective health-care reform: a reform in which the individual takes charge of his or her own body, and keeps that body in a state of exquisite good health.

Make no mistake: I'm not just talking about "wellness"—the buzzword that's come to mean so much in health-care circles. Wellness is really nothing more than the absence of disease. The Zone is beyond wellness. The Zone is about *optimal health*.

So how do we reach the Zone? Until now, the people who knew the most about it—the sports psychologists and trainers who work with elite athletes—have used a variety of techniques, including meditation, breathing exercises, visualization, and relaxation. Many of these tactics have been adopted not only from conventional Western psychology but from Far Eastern religious concepts and martial-arts training. But when these techniques do help the athlete reach the Zone, it's often by accident and can't be repeated with any degree of consistency.

So if psychology is at best a haphazard way to reach the Zone, what about pharmacology—that is, drugs? Among elite athletes looking for a competitive edge, the widespread use of performance-enhancing drugs, especially anabolic steroids and growth hormone, as well as practices such as blood doping, are well documented. But potentially there is a very high price to pay for a drug-enhanced performance edge—like your life.

Neither psychology nor drugs are a reliable way to get to the Zone. Sometimes they work, most often they don't.

There is only one route to reach the Zone at will. This technique will allow you not only to reach the Zone but to remain there throughout the day—and for weeks and months on end. This technique involves using the most powerful and ubiquitous drug we have: food.

That's right: no magic potions, pills, herbs, or mantras. The truth is that *every time you open your mouth to eat, you're applying for a passport to the Zone*. To get that passport, though, you must treat food as if it were a drug. You must eat food in a controlled fashion and in the proper proportions—as if it were an intravenous drip. Reaching the Zone is a matter of technology. It is based on principles of drug delivery that I've developed over the course of my career as a research scientist.

With computers, if you hit the correct key strokes, the wonders of that technology unfold. Hit the wrong keys, and the computer simply blinks at you. The dietary technology required to reach the Zone is as precise as any computer technology.

The rules of this dietary technology may appear complicated at first, but I think once you put them into practice you'll find they're exceptionally easy to follow. And like learning to use a computer, reaching the Zone requires following a defined set of rules.

The trouble is that most of us are using the wrong rules—eating the wrong foods, or, just as bad, eating the right foods in the wrong proportions. So our access to the Zone is being constantly denied. But follow the rules and your entrance is ensured. It's science.

What will you gain by following these rules? You'll get the background and the tools necessary to reach the Zone. If you follow the rules and stay within the boundaries of this dietary technology, you'll soon become a permanent resident. The rewards of increased energy, vitality, and performance—in work, in play, in personal relationships—will amaze you.

If this sounds like New Age jargon, it's not. It's the application of twenty-first-century biotechnology solutions to a twentieth-century problem—how to increase the efficiency of the human body.

THE REWARDS OF THE ZONE

Let me be a little more specific about the rewards you'll reap from staying in the Zone. One is loss of excess body fat. If you have a weight problem, the real problem is excess body fat. Even if you're only slightly overweight, the dietary technology I present in this book will help you lose that excess body fat and keep it off. You'll find that to be true even if every diet or lifestyle program you've ever tried has been a major disappointment. Just as important, you'll finally understand why traditional diets don't work. You weren't at fault; the diets you followed were in basic violation of the rules required to get to the Zone.

If being overweight—or having an unfortunate family history like mine—has you concerned about heart disease, this book will present great news. Over the past few years this dietary technology has been used to successfully treat patients suffering from *cardiomyopathy*, a tragic and potentially fatal form of heart disease. In this disease, the heart muscle gradually fails, so that the heart's ability to pump blood is compromised. Eventually, cardiomyopathy patients develop congestive heart failure—their hearts simply give out. There's no real treatment for this disease; patients who have it are usually given a terrible choice: get a heart transplant or die.

Steve Courson was one such patient. In the late 1970s, Steve was one of the strongest and most feared linemen in the National Football League, playing on two of the Pittsburgh Steelers' Super Bowl teams. In 1989, at the age of thirty-three, he was stricken with cardio-myopathy. He became so chronically fatigued that simple tasks such as climbing a flight of stairs were now extreme challenges. His chances of survival were considered so poor that he was put on a heart transplant list in the hopes that an acceptable donor would become available before his own heart gave out.

In the meantime, Steve was restricted from virtually all physical activity. For the next three years he was given a wide range of experi-mental drugs to keep his heart functioning. His condition failed to improve. His weight ballooned to more than 330 pounds. Taking out the garbage was now a major task for a man who only a few years earlier had taken on entire NFL defensive lines.

In 1992, Jon Kolb, an ex-Steeler teammate of Steve's, who was then the Steelers' strength coach, introduced Steve to me. When I explained to him the potential benefits of a Zone-favorable diet, he was interested but highly skeptical. He was also desperate, since after three years of treatment by the best of the Pittsburgh medical estab-lishment, he wasn't getting any better.

Steve faithfully followed the rules of the Zone-favorable technol-ogy. Within eighteen months he made a remarkable, almost miracu-lous transformation. His weight returned to his normal 260 pounds, and his percentage of body fat was now actually lower than it had been during his NFL days. His strength returned. His endurance ca-pacity, which had declined so drastically that he had become a virtual invalid, was now 50 percent greater than that of a normal person his age—even though he still had a compromised heart. Best of all, he was taken off the heart-transplant list. He got married, and is now looking forward to living a normal life span.

Steve's story is unusual, in that cardiomyopathy is a relatively unusual form of heart disease. But if following a Zone-favorable die-tary technology can help someone with cardiomyopathy, think what it can do for more common heart conditions—atherosclerosis, high blood pressure (hypertension), and high cholesterol (hypercholes-terolemia).

There's more. Using this Zone-favorable technology helps keep insulin levels on an even keel, so it's useful in treating diabetes. As an example, take Dr. Chris Kyriazis.

When Chris retired from IBM to live in Palm Desert, California, he should have been a very happy man. After all, as head of European marketing for IBM, he had had twenty thousand people working for him, and he had helped orchestrate his company's dominance of the European market.

But Chris's "golden years" weren't so golden. Not only had he developed diabetes, but he had high blood pressure; he'd already had a heart attack and was stricken with kidney cancer. "In 1992," he wrote me later, "my weight was 265 pounds, my blood pressure without medication was 220/120, my blood sugar was over 200 mg/dl, my right kidney had been removed because of cancer, and my left kidney showed signs of abnormal cells."

Today, after two years on a Zone-favorable diet, Chris writes: "My weight is 176 pounds, my blood pressure is 125/75 without taking any medication, my blood sugar is 70-90 mg/dl, I have no sign of my previous diabetic retinopathy, and my remaining kidney is free of any sign of cancer. Together with my family, I thank you for renewing my life's passport. My gratitude . . . runs very deep indeed."

Heart disease and diabetes are two of our country's most serious health problems. But the benefits of my Zone-favorable technology don't stop there. Reaching the Zone has a positive impact on a host of other disease states, including arthritis, and even "mental" diseases like depression and alcoholism. It can dramatically relieve chronic fatigue and restore energy, especially if you have chronic fatigue syndrome (CFS), premenstrual syndrome (PMS) or even HIV infection. And there are good theoretical reasons to believe that this dietary technology I've developed can be your best defense against cancer, not only by preventing its occurrence, but also by making tumors more vulnerable to attack by our bodies' own natural defenses, thereby increasing the effectiveness of anti-cancer drugs.

Of course, conditions such as heart disease, cancer, and diabetes are only one side—the dark side—of the story. The brighter side is the kind of maximum physical performance, better health and mental capacity that can be attained by entering and staying in the Zone.

As an example, let's take the swim teams at Stanford University. The coaches, Richard Quick for the women and Skip Kenney for the men, are considered among the finest in the world. They pride themselves on being at the cutting edge of elite athletic performance.

Introduced by a mutual friend, I told the Stanford coaches about my work with the Zone and its application to heart patients. They were intrigued by the possibility that a Zone-favorable diet could improve the performance of their athletes. With the 1992 Olympics approaching, they asked me if I would work with their swimmers.

The rest is history. At the Barcelona Olympics, Stanford swimmers won eight gold medals. Since that time both the men's and women's teams have dominated American swimming, winning the NCAA Swimming Championships in 1992, 1993, and 1994.

But most important, the quality of life for Richard and Skip has also improved. They both tell me that they have more energy, greater mental focus, and a greater sense of calm in a very high-pressure, demanding vocation. As Richard says, "I can't imagine anyone ever wanting to exit the Zone and return to life the way it used to be."

Richard has hit the nail on the head: living in the Zone should ultimately help *all* of us reach that most universal of personal goals—to live longer, healthier, and more satisfying lives.

OVERTURNING THE CURRENT WISDOM

The way we eat—or, at least, expert recommendations as to how we *should* eat—can be as much a matter of fad and fashion as the clothes we buy or the way we wear our hair. As with other fashions, notions about correct and healthful diet are constantly changing. Yesterday's dietary "laws" often become today's taboos.

For the past fifteen years or so, the reigning dietary "wisdom"—espoused by government nutrition boards, scientific panels, and private practitioners alike—has called for diets that are low in fat, low in protein, and high in carbohydrates. This formula has become dominant enough to produce dozens of best-selling variations on the theme, and to fill our supermarket shelves with hundreds of low-fat, high-carb products—not to mention filling us with guilt and anxiety when we don't eat as we're told. Worse yet, with these diets we often get fatter even while following their guidelines with religious fervor.

Low fat, low protein, high carbohydrate: that's the current wisdom in today's dietary marketplace. Well, let's say it plainly: *much of the current wisdom is dead wrong*. In fact, if you follow the more extreme of today's fashionable low-fat, low-protein, high-carbohydrate diets, you may actually be putting yourself in danger.

If you're overweight, you'll be doomed to stay that way. Even worse, following some of these trendy diets can actually increase your risk of contracting serious and even life-threatening diseases. This book is meant as a corrective, an antidote to the well-meaning but misguided dietary advice that's not only keeping you fat but also keeping you from enjoying maximum good health.

Confusion and frustration are leading Americans to become fearful of food; whatever they eat, they seem to become worse off. People desperately want to believe that diet is the best way to a healthier and more productive life. That's what I want to deliver in this book: a newer, simpler, and better way to eat, based on science, not intuition—a road map to a new and better you. Why make life more difficult than it has to be? Life is much more enjoyable in the Zone.

In Chapter 8 you'll find the diet: the key to living in the nearly euphoric metabolic state called the Zone. In this program, food is used to maintain a favorable hormonal balance, especially among insulin, glucagon and the superhormones called eicosanoids.

The following chapters explain why all that is true—that and much more. Those of you who want to get started right away and learn how and what to eat may want to skip ahead to Chapter 8 and return later for the explanation.

CHAPTER TWO

THE FATTENING OF AMERICA

You fatten cattle by feeding them lots and lots of low-fat grain. How do you fatten humans? Same way: you feed them lots and lots of low-fat grain. So if you've been eating more pasta and bread (both made from grain) than ever before, and you're still gaining weight, think about those grain-fed cattle the next time you sit down to a big plate of pasta.

THE GREAT CARBOHYDRATE EXPERIMENT

For the past fifteen years, the people of this country have been unwitting participants in a massive scientific experiment. The goal of that experiment was exceptionally noble—the reduction of excess body fat in the American population. If such a goal was attainable, our healthier population would dramatically decrease the burdens on the existing health-care system, especially for an aging population. (By conservative estimates, the cost of treating conditions related to obesity in 1986 was $39 billion.)

But how to achieve that goal? The message, from top scientists, nutritionists, and the government, was simple: Americans were told to eat less fat and more carbohydrates. That, said the experts, is how you get skinnier. *complex*

We're now fifteen years into the experiment, and one doesn't have to be a rocket scientist to see that it isn't working. In fact, all data analysis during the last fifteen years of this experiment shows that in spite of the fact that the American public has dramatically cut back on the amount of fat consumed, the country has experienced an epidemic rise in obesity. *eating sugars (+ fats, still)*

The sad truth is that Americans are getting fatter. A recent study by scientists at the National Center for Health Statistics in the Centers for Disease Control and Prevention showed that the number of overweight adults in America—one-quarter of the population from 1960 to 1980—suddenly jumped between 1980 and 1991 to one-*third* of the population. That's a 32 percent increase in obesity in just ten years. If there were a 32 percent increase in heart disease or a 32 percent increase in breast cancer in a similar time period, it would be a national emergency. (Actually, as I'll show later, within another ten to twenty years this increase in obesity is likely to manifest itself in similar increases in those disease states as well.)

Researchers at the National Institutes of Health recently revealed that during the last seven years, while the dietary intake of saturated fats and cholesterol was decreasing, the average weight of young adult Americans has actually *increased* by ten pounds!

"Shocking," said the experts who conducted the study. "Totally unexpected." And indeed it's obvious that something is very wrong. If we're eating supposedly "healthy" diets that supply less fat and less cholesterol, why in the world are we gaining weight?

That straightforward question has a straight answer: we're getting fatter because many of our dietary "laws" are wrong.

In addition, many of today's fashionable recommendations are confusing. If you read enough of these low-fat, high-carbohydrate dietary formulas, you'll find little agreement—even among the scientific experts—as to precise definitions for "low" and "high."

The National Research Council's prestigious Committee on Diet and Health, for example, recommends that most Americans get 30 percent of their total daily calories from fats, and 55 percent or more from carbohydrates—especially so-called "complex" carbohydrates like pasta and bread. That's one set of recommendations.

But when *Consumer Reports* magazine—a highly respected, even authoritative publication—asked a panel of sixty-eight scientific experts on nutrition (some of whom sit on the NRC Committee on Diet and Health), they got a different answer. The panel assembled by *Consumer Reports* recommended limiting fat intake to as little as twenty percent of daily calories, and a vague "more than half" of daily calories from carbohydrates.

And protein? The National Research Council Committee tells you to "maintain protein intake at moderate levels." What's a moderate level? Who knows? Meanwhile, the *Consumer Reports* panel says, "Don't worry about protein one way or the other. Most Americans eat at least as much protein as they need."

These differences are confounding people who want a simple, standard set of figures. But the confusion's just starting. The National Research Council's committee and the *Consumer Reports* panel represent the conservative end of what is actually a wide spectrum of low-fat, high-carb recommendations. At the other end of the spectrum are the people I think of as the low-fat radicals. Led by the late Nathan Pritikin, author of *The Pritikin Program for Diet and Exercise*, these dietary extremists advocate that only 5 to 10 percent of total calories should come from fats, 10 to 15 percent from protein, and a whopping 75 to 85 percent from carbohydrates.

No wonder the average American is confused.

But the confusion caused by these conflicting recommendations is only one problem. The greater problem is the terrible paradox: people are eating less fat and getting fatter! No medical authority will tell you that excess body fat makes you healthier. There is but one alarming conclusion to reach: a high-carbohydrate, low-fat diet may be dangerous to your health.

To understand why that is, we need a new perspective on food. We need to understand the relationship between the food we eat and our potential to live in the Zone. If you're not in the Zone, one major consequence may be the relentless accumulation of excess body fat— even with an almost fat-free diet.

To get a new perspective on food, here's some information you need to know. Some of it may surprise you.

• *Eating fat does not make you fat.* It's your body's response to excess carbohydrates in your diet that makes you fat. Your body has a limited capacity to store excess carbohydrates, but it can easily convert those excess carbohydrates into excess body fat.

• *It's hard to lose weight by simply restricting calories.* Eating less and losing excess body fat do not automatically go hand in hand. Low-calorie, high-carbohydrate diets generate a series of biochemical signals in your body that will take you out of the Zone, making it more difficult to access stored body fat for energy. Result: you'll reach a weight-loss plateau, beyond which you simply can't lose any more weight.

• *Diets based on choice restriction and calorie limits usually fail.* People on restrictive diets get tired of feeling hungry and deprived.

They go off their diets, put the weight back on (primarily as increased body fat), and then feel bad about themselves for not having enough will power, discipline, or motivation.

• *Weight loss has little to do with will power.* You need information, not will power. If you change *what* you eat, you don't have to be overly concerned about *how much* you eat. Adhering to a diet of Zone-favorable meals, you can eat enough to feel satisfied and still wind up losing fat—without obsessively counting calories or fat grams.

• *Food can be good or bad.* The ratio of macronutrients—protein, carbohydrate, and fat—in the meals you eat is the key to permanent weight loss and optimal health. Unless you understand the rules that control the powerful biochemical responses generated by food, you will never reach the Zone.

• *The biochemical effects of food have been constant for the last forty million years.* All mammals, including man, have essentially the same responses to food. These responses have been genetically conserved throughout evolution, and are unlikely to change in the near future.

Bottom line: the key to losing fat is not a matter of cutting calories, it's a matter of reaching the Zone. In the Zone losing body fat is virtually automatic. But to reach the Zone and stay there on a permanent basis, you'll first need to understand the difference between weight loss and fat loss.

FAT LOSS VERSUS WEIGHT LOSS

Nutrition, like religion, is extremely visceral. For many people, it's a matter of faith that a pound lost is a pound lost, and it doesn't really matter where that lost weight came from. So let me make something clear: there's a big difference between weight loss and fat loss.

Obesity is not simply weight gain. It's the accumulation of *excess* body fat. Thus, reaching an ideal body weight is not just a matter of losing weight. It involves the reduction of *excess* body fat.

Your body weight is composed of many factors—water content, fat content, muscle content, and structural component (bones, tendons, etc.). For simplicity, though, you can treat the body as a two-part system: pure fat on the one hand, and lean body mass (everything else) on the other. Your percentage of body fat is simply your total fat content divided by your total weight (Total Fat ÷ Total Body Weight = % Body Fat).

When you want to calculate your *ideal* body weight, you're not looking for some mystical number. Your ideal body weight is simply the appropriate percent of body fat for a healthy male or female. That figure is usually accepted to be 15 percent body fat for males and 22 percent body fat for females. (The higher amount of body fat for females is a reflection of the genetic differences between men and women.)

(The old Metropolitan Life Tables for ideal body weight—which have consistently revised upwards over the years and which almost no one in America comes close to matching—are included in Appendix G.)

How do current Americans stack up in terms of body fat? Today's average American man has 23 percent body fat, while the average American woman has 32 percent body fat. This means the average male in this country is 53 percent fatter than his ideal, and the average female 50 percent fatter than hers. Americans are without question the fattest people on the face of the planet.

Why are our body-fat percentages so high? Because the experts who are telling us what to eat don't really understand the relationship between diet and fat loss. Specifically, the experts don't quite understand how body fat is influenced by the *macronutrient* content of the food we eat.

What are macronutrients? Very simple: protein, carbohydrates, and fat.

This concept may seem mundane. Of course food consists of protein, carbohydrates, and fat—you've been told that since the fourth grade. But the truth goes much deeper. The fact is that every time you eat these macronutrients generate complex hormonal responses in your body. These responses ultimately determine how much body fat you will store. In terms of weight loss, knowing how to control these responses is the real power of nutrition, and hence the gateway to the Zone.

So let's take a look at the macronutrients, one by one:

CARBOHYDRATES—THE REASON YOU'RE FAT

Over the past fifteen years, our dietary establishment has made a virtual industry of extolling the virtues of carbohydrates. We're constantly told that carbohydrates are the good guys of nutrition, and that, if we eat large amounts of them, the world should be a better place. In such a world, the experts tell us, there will be no heart disease and no obesity. Under such guidance, Americans are gobbling breads, cereals, and pastas as if there were no tomorrow, trying desperately to reach that 80 to 85 percent of total calories advocated by the high-carb extremists.

Unfortunately, many people don't really know what a carbohydrate is. Most people will say carbohydrates are sweets and pasta. Ask them what a vegetable or fruit is, and they'll probably reply that it's a vegetable or fruit—as if that were a food type all its own, a food type that they can eat in unlimited amounts without gaining weight.

Well, this may come as a surprise, but all of the above—sweets and pasta, vegetables and fruits—are carbohydrates. Carbohydrates are merely different forms of simple sugars linked together in polymers—something like edible plastic.

Of course, we all need a certain amount of carbohydrates in our diet. The body requires a continual intake of carbohydrates to feed the brain, which uses glucose (a form of sugar) as its primary energy source. In fact, the brain is a virtual glucose hog, gobbling more than two thirds of the circulating carbohydrates in the bloodstream while you are at rest. To feed this glucose hog, the body continually takes carbohydrates and converts them to glucose.

It's actually a bit more complicated than that. Any carbohydrates not immediately used by the body will be stored in the form of glycogen (a long string of glucose molecules linked together). The body has two storage sites for glycogen: the liver and the muscles. The glycogen stored in the muscles is inaccessible to the brain. Only the glycogen stored in the liver can be broken down and sent back to the bloodstream so as to maintain adequate blood sugar levels for proper brain function.

The liver's capacity to store carbohydrates in the form of glycogen is very limited and can be easily depleted within ten to twelve hours. So the liver's glycogen reserves must be maintained on a continual basis. That's why we eat carbohydrates.

The question no one has bothered to ask until now is this: what happens when you eat *too much* carbohydrate? Here's the answer: whether it's being stored in the liver or the muscles, the total storage capacity of the body for carbohydrate is really quite limited. If you're an average person, you can store about three hundred to four hundred grams of carbohydrate in your muscles, but you can't get at that carbohydrate. In the liver, where carbohydrates are accessible for glucose conversion, you can store only about sixty to ninety grams. This is equivalent to about two cups of cooked pasta or three typical candy bars, and it represents your total reserve capacity to keep the brain working properly.

Once the glycogen levels are filled in both the liver and the muscles, excess carbohydrates have just one fate: to be converted into fat and stored in the adipose, that is, fatty, tissue. In a nutshell, even though carbohydrates themselves are fat-free, *excess carbohydrates end up as excess fat.*

That's not the worst of it. Any meal or snack *high* in carbohydrates will generate a rapid rise in blood glucose. To adjust for this rapid rise, the pancreas secretes the hormone insulin into the bloodstream. Insulin then lowers the levels of blood glucose.

All well and good. The problem is that insulin is essentially a storage hormone, evolved to put aside excess carbohydrate calories in the form of fat in case of future famine. So the insulin that's stimulated by excess carbohydrates aggressively promotes the accumulation of body fat.

In other words, when we eat too much carbohydrate, we're essentially sending a hormonal message, via insulin, to the body (actually, to the adipose cells). The message: "Store fat."

Hold on; it gets even worse. Not only do increased insulin levels tell the body to store carbohydrates as fat, they also tell it not to release any stored fat. This makes it impossible for you to use your own stored body fat for energy. So the excess carbohydrates in your diet not only make you fat, they make sure you *stay* fat. It's a double whammy, and it can be lethal.

To put it another way, too much carbohydrate means too much insulin, and too much insulin takes you out of the Zone. Out of the

Zone, you put on excess body fat, and you can't get rid of it.

That's the carbohydrate picture in outline. Let's sharpen the focus. The real key to all this is the speed at which carbohydrates enter the bloodstream, because that's what controls the rate of insulin secretion. You see, the stomach is basically an indiscriminate vat of acid that takes all carbohydrates—whether they're puffed-rice cakes, refined table sugar, carrots, or pasta—and breaks them down into simple sugars for absorption. What distinguishes one kind of carbohydrate from another is the rate at which the carbohydrate enters the bloodstream.

Before 1980 no one bothered to ask about the entry rates into the bloodstream of various types of carbohydrates. When this question was finally studied, the implications should have turned the nutritional community on its head. Somehow supposedly "simple" sugars like fructose were entering the bloodstream at far slower rates than supposedly "complex" carbohydrates like pasta. This fact has major consequences if you ever hope to reach the Zone.

The entry rate of a carbohydrate into the bloodstream is known as its *glycemic index*. The lower the glycemic index, the slower the rate of absorption. Believe it or not, refined table sugar has a lower glycemic index than typical breakfast cereals. Actually, the carbohydrate that turned out to have one of the highest glycemic indices—that is, the fastest recorded entry rates into the bloodstream—was the basic centerpiece of many weight-reduction programs: puffed-rice cakes. In fact, puffed-rice cakes have a much higher glycemic index than ice cream, which is supposed to be the weight watcher's worst enemy.

Say it ain't so.

What determines the glycemic index? The primary factors are (1) the structure of the simple sugars in the food, (2) the soluble fiber content, and (3) the fat content. I'll come back to the fat content in a moment; for now let's talk about the other two.

How does the structure of the simple sugar that makes up the carbohydrate affect the sugar's rate of entry into the bloodstream? Remember that all "complex" carbohydrates must be broken down into simple sugars for absorption. There are only three common sugars that comprise all edible carbohydrates, and each one has a different molecular structure, which ultimately determines its rate of entry into the bloodstream. Glucose is the most common of these sugars, followed by fructose and galactose.

Glucose is found in grains, pasta, bread, cereals, starches, and vegetables. Fructose is primarily found in fruits. Galactose is found in dairy products. However, while all of these simple sugars are rapidly absorbed by the liver, only glucose can be released directly into the bloodstream. This is why glucose-rich carbohydrates like breads and pasta virtually sprint from the liver back into the bloodstream, while galactose and fructose, which must first be converted to glucose in the liver, enter the bloodstream at a slower rate.

For fructose especially, this a very slow process. That's why even though they're primarily made up of simple sugars, fructose-containing carbohydrates (primarily fruits), have a very low glycemic index compared to glucose and galactose-containing carbohydrates.

What about the fiber content? Fiber (which is nondigestible carbohydrate) is not absorbed, and therefore it has no effect on insulin directly. However, it does act as a brake on the rate of entry on the absorption of other carbohydrates into the bloodstream. The higher the fiber content of a carbohydrate, the slower the rate of entry into the bloodstream. Remove the fiber of the carbohydrate and the rate of entry accelerates. So fiber is a significant factor in controlling the speed at which the body absorbs carbohydrate. In effect, fiber acts as a control rod to prevent a runaway rate of carbohydrate absorption. (This, by the way, is the same reason that there are control rods in nuclear reactors—to prevent potentially dangerous runaway reactions.)

That's why the recent popularity of juicing (the removal of fiber from fruits to make easy-to-drink juices) has been a disaster. Juicing simply removes a primary control rod (i.e., fiber) from the carbohydrate, meaning that the carbohydrate enters the bloodstream too fast.

When a carbohydrate enters the bloodstream too fast, the pancreas responds by secreting high levels of insulin. While that brings the blood-sugar level down, it also tells the body to store fat and keep it stored.

So too many high-glycemic carbohydrates can not only make you fat, they will also keep you that way. A complete listing of the glycemic index of carbohydrates is given in Appendix H; you can use these simple rules to determine whether a carbohydrate's glycemic index is high or low. Virtually all fruits (except bananas and dried fruits) and virtually all fiber-rich vegetables (except carrots and corn) are low-glycemic carbohydrates. Virtually all grains, starches, and pasta are high-glycemic carbohydrates.

Ironically, high-glycemic carbohydrates like grains, breads, and pasta are the base of the new and supposedly healthy "food pyramid" established by the U.S. government. Yet these are precisely the types of carbohydrates that promote increased insulin secretion, and, as you've found out, higher insulin levels make you fat.

So if you're trying to lose weight, eating too many carbohydrates, especially high-glycemic carbohydrates—and the resulting increase in insulin levels—can have exactly the wrong effect. Instead of burning off your stockpiles of stored fat, you're actually increasing them. Instead of getting leaner, you're getting fatter.

The next time you reach for a fat-free puffed-rice cake, you may want to keep that in mind.

PROTEIN—THE NEGLECTED MACRONUTRIENT

If carbohydrates are the good-guy macronutrients in contemporary nutritional mythology, the two bad guys are fats and proteins. Let's take proteins first. The justification for protein's bad rap is that two of our most popular protein sources, red meat and whole dairy products, also contain large amounts of saturated fats. These fats can be unhealthy.

But instead of simply restricting the amounts of these two *types* of protein, some of today's trendy diets tend to lump *all* types of protein together and restrict them all. This is a case of throwing out the baby with the bath water. Protein's recent bad reputation—and the restrictive dietary recommendations that accompany it—is a misleading overreaction.

Proteins are the basis of all life. In our bodies, protein is more plentiful than any other substance but water. As much as one-half of your dry body weight—including most of your muscle mass, skin, hair, eyes, and nails—is made up of protein.

Protein is the main structural ingredient of our cells, and the enzymes that keep them running. Even our immune systems are essentially composed of protein. Amino acids, the building blocks of protein, are the foundation of all life.

There are twenty of these vital amino acids. Nine of them, known as the essential amino acids, cannot be synthesized by the human body, and must be supplied by the diet. Without these essential amino acids constantly entering the body, the rates of new protein formation will slow down, and in the extreme case stop altogether. You can see why having adequate levels of protein on a daily basis is critical. You must constantly provide the building blocks for new protein formation. Without bricks, you can't have walls.

All right, if protein is a necessary fact of life—and if excess carbohydrate makes you fat—why not eat lots of protein and very little carbohydrate? Wouldn't that help you lose that excess body fat?

In fact, high-protein, low-carbohydrate diets are the basis of many quick weight-loss programs, whether they're sold over the counter or medically supervised. The typical slogan of these programs: "Eat all the protein you want and all the fat you want, just cut back on the carbohydrates."

At first glance, these quick-loss programs look good. Almost everyone who tries them does lose weight at first. Unfortunately, those people are losing the wrong kind of weight, and for the wrong biological reasons.

The truth is that these high-protein, quick-loss diets induce an abnormal metabolic state known as *ketosis*. This occurs when you have insufficient carbohydrate stored in the liver to meet the requirements of the body and the brain. (Remember that even when "full" the liver stores only small amounts of carbohydrate.) Once that stored carbohydrate is used up, which takes less than twenty-four hours on a low-carbohydrate diet, the body turns to fat to supply energy. Great, you say—isn't that what we want?

Unfortunately, with a high-protein, low-carbohydrate diet, that's often not what you get. The process of converting fat into energy gets short-circuited on a low-carbohydrate, ketogenic diet. As a result, your cells manufacture abnormal biochemicals called *ketone bodies*.

The body has no use for these ketone bodies. It tries like mad to get rid of them through increased urination. That spells weight loss—at first—but the vast bulk of that weight loss is merely water. That high-protein diet hasn't really touched most of your excess body fat.

These high-protein, quick-weight-loss programs have you losing the wrong kind of weight. And that's not even the worst of it. If you eat too much protein at a meal, your insulin levels will also start to increase because your body doesn't want a lot of excess amino acids floating around in the bloodstream. What will the increased insulin levels do? They now help convert the excess protein into fat.

It's also been discovered recently that high-protein, ketogenic diets may cause changes in the fat cells, making them ten times more active in sequestering fat than they were before you went on the diet. So when you go off the diet, you continue to accumulate fat at a frightening rate. (This is commonly known as the "yo-yo syndrome.")

Add insult to injury. The body isn't stupid. When it has to deal with a high-protein, low-carbohydrate diet, it says, "Hey, I didn't fall off the turnip truck. The brain needs carbohydrate to function, so I'll start ripping down muscle mass, and I'll turn much of the protein in that muscle mass into carbohydrate." You might say, "That's fine; I can live with losing some muscle until I lose my body fat." But remember: because of those increased insulin levels, you're not losing fat at anywhere near the rate you expect, and you eventually reach a weight plateau.

Put all this together, and you'll see why more than 95 percent of the people who have ever lost weight using high-protein, ketogenic diets have gained that weight back and more. Why? Is everyone who ever tried a quick-weight-loss program a weak-willed ninny? I don't think so. It's just that their high-protein, low-carbohydrate diets have caused permanent changes in their fat cells, changes that virtually guarantee increased body-fat accumulation in the future.

FAT PHOBIA

What's the most feared three-letter word in the American dietary dictionary? F-A-T. Nowhere in the world is fat phobia more extreme than in the United States and nowhere else are people fatter. While Americans think of carbohydrates as the savior of mankind, fat is considered the messenger of doom.

I've said it before and I'll say it again: *dietary fat does not make you fat.* What's more—and this is even more shocking—*you have to eat fat to lose fat.*

This sounds like nutritional heresy, but there's scientific proof. In the 1950s, Kekwick and Pawan at the University of London in England published a landmark study. They put patients on a diet that was low in calories (1,000 calories) but high in fat. In fact, fat supplied 90 percent of the total calories. What happened? *Those patients lost significant amounts of weight.* When the same patients were put on a high-carbohydrate diet (90 percent of the calories as carbohydrate) with the same number of calories, *there was virtually no weight loss.* Amazing.

There's further proof, closer to home. Remember that currently trendy high-carbohydrate diets are keeping people fat, *even though the fat content of these diets is very low.* With the Zone-favorable diet I've developed, the fat content is exceptionally important: in fact, it's the biochemical key that ultimately prevents the accumulation of excess body fat. In other words, in a Zone-favorable diet *you use fat to lose fat.*

So what happens when overweight people go on a Zone-favorable diet that combines the proper ratios of protein, carbohydrate, and fat? In 1992 I conducted a pilot study to answer this question. In this study, I used 91 people—63 women and 28 men—age 25 to 55. All these people were healthy and normal, but slightly overweight. (The average percent of body fat was 29 percent for the women and 20 percent for the men—less body fat than average Americans of the same sex, but still more than the ideal.) These were classic Americans: people who have five to ten extra pounds that they can't seem to lose no matter how much they diet or exercise. As you can imagine, it wasn't too hard to recruit such a group of test subjects.

What did I expect? A weight loss of about one pound per week. (It's genetically impossible to lose more than 1 to 1½ pounds of body fat per week—you just can't lose body fat any faster. You can lose more weight, but that will be primarily water loss and muscle-mass loss. That's why people on quick weight loss programs look so haggard—they're losing muscle mass.)

First, I determined the daily protein requirement for each person in the study. (As I'll show later, this protein requirement is unique for each individual.) Then I had each person eat three meals and two snacks a day. Each meal and snack contained the appropriate amounts of protein, carbohydrates, and fat to get into the Zone. To induce compliance, I also developed an experimental prototype food bar (that looked and tasted like a candy bar) with the correct macronutrient composition needed to enter the Zone. I had the study volunteers use the bars as a meal replacement for breakfast.

The results of this six-week study (shown in Table 2-1) were exactly as I expected: the women lost an average of seven pounds of fat, a little more than one pound of fat per week. There was no loss of lean body mass, so all of the weight loss was pure fat loss. Their average percentage of body fat dropped from 29 percent to 26 percent—a reduction of 11 percent from their starting body-fat percentage.

Now for the statistical analysis. Statistics tell you the likelihood of doing the same experiment and getting the same results. A statistically significant experiment in science is one in which the results can be replicated 95 times out of 100 (this would represent a p factor of less than 0.05). The *p factor* is the probability that the results are due to chance. The lower the p factor, the greater the likelihood of reproducing the same results in another similar experiment. This p factor gives a pretty good indication that your result is not due to random chance.

What were the statistics for this pilot weight-loss study in the women? They were great: the p factor was less than 0.0005. In essence, the statistics said that if you repeated the same study 10,000 times, you'd get the same results 9,995 times.

TABLE 2-1

Pilot Fat Loss in Slightly Overweight Individuals

PARAMETER	STARTING	ENDING	CHANGE	SIGNIFICANCE
Women (n = 63)				
Weight (lbs.)	159	153	–6	P < 0.0005
Fat mass (lbs.)	48	41	–7	P < 0.0005
Lean mass (lbs.)	111	112	+1	P < 0.05
Percent body fat	29	26	–3	P < 0.0005
Men (n = 28)				
Weight (lbs.)	195	192	–3	P < 0.25
Fat mass (lbs.)	40	33	–7	P < 0.0005
Lean mass (lbs.)	155	158	+3	P < 0.005
Percent body fat	20	17	–3	P < 0.0005

The men did just as well—they also lost body fat while increasing their lean body mass simultaneously. The increase in lean body mass for the men meant that their total weight loss was not statistically significant. But their fat loss and decrease in percent of body fat were statistically highly significant. In fact, their percentage of body fat dropped from 20 percent to 17 percent. This was a 15 percent reduction from the percentage of starting body fat, very similar to the 11 percent found for the women. Like the women, the statistics predicted the same result would be achieved 9,995 times out of 10,000.

More important, neither the men nor the women lost any lean body (muscle) mass. All the weight loss was fat loss. What's the bottom line? Even if you've failed on every other weight-loss program, these statistics say that if you follow a Zone-favorable diet, you're likely to succeed.

Keep in mind the two keys to permanent weight loss through a Zone-favorable diet: (1) dietary fat does not make you fat; and (2) you have to eat fat to lose fat. Yes, this flies in the face of everything you've ever been told about diet and weight loss, and yes, it will be explained.

It's really quite simple: it comes down to how your hormones respond to the food you eat. The more you know about these responses, the more likely you'll get to the Zone. And once you're in the Zone, your weight worries will become a thing of the past.

But the door swings both ways. The hormonal responses generated by the food you eat can be your greatest ally, or your worst nightmare.

CHAPTER THREE

THE HORMONAL EFFECTS OF FOOD

Say the word *hormone*, and most people immediately think of sex. And certainly the so-called "sex hormones"—testosterone and estrogen—have vital jobs to do, not just in regulating sexual drive but in maintaining good health in general.

Important as they are, testosterone and estrogen are but two soldiers in the vast army of hormones that come as standard equipment in all living organisms. Yet few of us realize how crucial hormones really are. The truth is that hormones regulate virtually everything your body does—from controlling blood-sugar levels to the basic survival mechanisms involved in stress, fear, and even love.

In many ways hormones can be viewed as your internal phone system, allowing distant parts of the body to communicate with speed and tight coordination. Like the phone system, you have three kinds of communication links: long distance, regional, and local.

The hormonal version of long-distance communication is known as the endocrine system. Endocrine hormones represent the classic type of hormonal responses, and can be viewed as the body's equivalent to a series of microwave towers or a fiber-optic network. Like these communication megastructures, endocrine hormones are relatively easy to study.

In the endocrine system, the action begins when a secreting gland sends a message in the form of a hormone into the bloodstream, which is the body's version of the fiber-optic network. The hormonal message travels through the bloodstream to reach a distant target cell. The cell receives the message and responds with the action that's been ordered by the hormonal messenger.

As an example of the power of the hormones in action, let's use insulin. The pancreas secretes insulin into the bloodstream. The insulin travels to the liver and to the muscle cells, telling them to take glucose from the bloodstream and store it. The liver and muscle cells do just that.

As insulin levels increase, blood-glucose levels begin to fall. Once blood glucose falls below a critical level, the brain, which needs glucose to function, begins to call out for more glucose. If the brain doesn't get the glucose it wants, it starts tuning out.

Medically, this glucose shortage is known as hypoglycemia or low blood sugar. When it happens to adults, it produces mental fatigue. That's why when you eat a big pasta meal at noon by three o'clock you can barely keep your eyes open. When this happens to athletes—and it happens even though they've been drinking carbohydrate-rich "energy" drinks during the race—it's called "bonking." When it happens to kids—as it does, for example, at a day-care center after the three-o'clock snack with apple juice—it's called total bedlam.

When hypoglycemia strikes, what prevents the liver from simply replenishing the blood glucose from its storage depot? The answer is high levels of insulin. The same exaggerated insulin response generated by that pasta lunch, or that high-carb sports drink, or that three-o'clock apple juice at the day-care center, now prevents the replenishment of blood glucose that supplies the brain with the fuel it needs. Now you start tuning out. As you can see, the effects of a long-distance endocrine hormone in action can be widespread and very potent.

In paracrine hormonal responses, the hormone travels only a very short distance from a secreting cell to a target cell. Because of the short distance between the secreting cell and the target cell, paracrine responses don't need the long-distance capabilities of the bloodstream. Instead, they use the body's version of a regional system: the paracrine system.

Finally, there are the autocrine hormone systems, analogous to the cord that links the handset of the phone to the phone itself. Here the secreting cells release a hormone that comes immediately back to affect the secreting cell itself.

The hormones in the paracrine and autocrine systems are short-acting, and are difficult to study because they don't appear in the bloodstream, where they can be easily sampled. They also tend to be even more powerful than endocrine hormones, working at much lower concentrations. Because of their powerful physiological actions, these hormones tend to self-destruct within seconds after accomplishing their task. The fleeting physiological effects of these paracrine and autocrine hormonal responses are a crucial part of the scientific foundation needed to understand how to enter the Zone.

The other feature of that scientific foundation is the fact that hormonal systems are constantly engaged in a balancing act. Hormones rarely act as lone rangers. The hormones in a given system are usually paired in sets (a set is called an *axis*), consisting of two hormones with powerful but totally opposite physiological effects.

There are many paired sets of endocrine hormones, but the most important in terms of reaching the Zone is the insulin-glucagon axis. Insulin drives down blood-sugar levels, while glucagon has the opposite effect: it increases blood-sugar levels. The balancing of these opposed physiological effects allows the body to maintain a relatively tight control of blood sugar, allowing the brain to function at its best. If this tight hormonal balance is disturbed, if the communication in the system breaks down, the result is an imbalance of blood-glucose levels.

If insulin levels are too high, for example, or if glucagon levels are too low, the result is hypoglycemia, or low blood sugar. When that happens, brain function is compromised. There is also a condition known as insulin resistance, in which insulin levels are elevated but blood-sugar levels remain high because the target cells no longer respond to insulin. Insulin resistance and the resulting *elevated insulin levels* (hyperinsulinemia) lead to the accumulation of excess body fat, and prolonged hyperinsulinemia can not only promote diabetes but also speed up the development of heart disease.

This is not just an academic discussion of hormonal biochemistry. It turns out that the food you eat has an exceptionally powerful effect on all these hormonal responses: endocrine, paracrine, and autocrine. Once you understand the power of the hormonal responses generated by the food you eat, you can no longer think of food simply as a source of calories for the body.

Any nutritionist can tell you how many grams of fat there are in a serving of food, or how many calories a meal provides. But optimal health is not a consequence of counting calories. It's based on an understanding of the complex hormonal responses that are generated every time you open your mouth to eat (see Figure 3-1). Once you understand these hormonal responses, many of the conceptions you have about human nutrition may be seen to be totally false.

If we use this hormonal point of view to look at a spectrum of conventional diets, we can see that for various and often different reasons all of them are doomed to fail. To put it another way, *all conventional weight reduction diets are hormonally incorrect*. No matter how well intentioned, they can't help you lose weight and keep it off permanently. They can't help prevent or treat disease, and they can't promote the optimal health and maximum performance that come once you're in the Zone.

The truth is that all conventional diets ignore one vital fact: *food is the most powerful drug you will ever encounter. Learning how to control hormonal responses to food is your passport to entering and staying in the Zone.*

How do you use food to control hormonal responses? You must begin by thinking of food not as a source of calories but as a control system for hormones. Think of the composition of each meal as a hormonal ATM card that will determine which energy source you are going to use for the next four to six hours. Hit the correct ATM code, and you tap into a virtually unlimited source of energy—your own stored body fat. Hit the wrong code, and you will be forced to use a fuel that's low octane and in limited supply: stored carbohydrates.

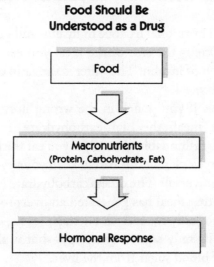

**Food Should Be
Understood as a Drug**

Food

⬇

Macronutrients
(Protein, Carbohydrate, Fat)

⬇

Hormonal Response

Figure 3-1

(The typical person has nearly 100,000 calories stored as body fat for potential energy. How many carbohydrate-loaded pancakes do you have to eat to give you the same amount of energy? The answer is a lot—about 1,700.)

That correct hormonal ATM code—your secret password for entering the Zone—lies hidden in the insulin-glucagon axis. Insulin, you'll recall, is a storage hormone. Its job is to take excess glucose from dietary carbohydrates and excess amino acids from dietary protein, and store them in the adipose tissues as fat. It's also helpful to think of insulin as a locking hormone: not only does it store fat in the adipose tissue, it locks that stored fat up so it can't be released.

If insulin is a storage and locking hormone, then glucagon, insulin's biological opposite, is a mobilization hormone. Glucagon's primary job is to release stored carbohydrates, in the form of glucose, from the liver. Once released by glucagon, this glucose enters the bloodstream, and helps maintain the tight balance of blood sugar required for the brain to function adequately.

Since insulin drives down blood sugar, and glucagon restores blood-sugar levels, the communication and ongoing balance of these two hormones is critical for survival. Remember that the release of insulin is stimulated by carbohydrates, especially by high-glycemic carbohydrates like breads and pastas. On the other hand, glucagon (which, like insulin, is secreted by the pancreas) is stimulated by dietary protein.

So the critical hormonal balance of insulin and glucagon depends on two things. One is the size of the meal you eat—excess calories stimulate secretion of insulin. The other is the ratio of protein to carbohydrate in each meal.

What happens if you punch in the wrong hormonal code—the typical big pasta meal, the high-carbohydrate, low-protein meal that's currently so fashionable? Usually if you eat the big pasta meal at twelve, by three o'clock you can barely keep your eyes open. Why is this response so universal? The excess carbohydrate (and lack of sufficient protein) in that meal has generated an overproduction of insulin. The insulin not only reduces blood-sugar levels—thereby depriving the brain of its only source of energy—but it also prevents the replenishment of blood sugar from the liver.

As blood-sugar levels drop, the brain begins to tune out. Within three to four hours after a high-carbohydrate meal, the brain is getting desperate for energy (even though you probably have the equivalent of two or three candy bars stored in your liver, desperate to get out). But this massive amount of stored carbohydrate can't be released into the bloodstream because the high-carbohydrate meal you ate drove insulin levels up and glucagon levels down.

Since glucagon levels remain low, you can't replenish blood sugar from your own internal stored carbohydrate in the liver. In desperation, your brain tells you that bag of corn chips looks very inviting. While eating the corn chips (or Oreo cookies) does supply an immediate source of carbohydrates for the brain, it simply restarts the vicious circle of raised insulin and diminished glucagon. In other words, you're stuck in carbohydrate hell.

Carbohydrate hell is the source of all your carbohydrate cravings—including the infamous sweet tooth—and the constant cycle of recurring hunger (every two to three hours) that goes with them. These cravings are hormonally driven by that high-carbohydrate meal—or, more accurately, by a macronutrient ratio that was too high in carbohydrate and too low in protein.

If carbohydrate cravings were the only result of punching up the

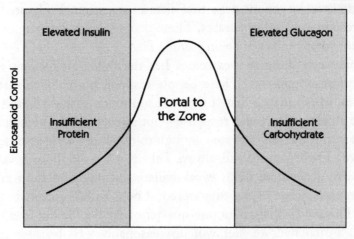

Figure 3-2

wrong hormonal code, that would be bad enough. Remember: your glycogen depots in the liver and muscles are stuffed full, but you're still eating carbohydrates. Where and how are you going to store the excess? That excess carbohydrate ends up being converted into fat. For fat, the body can always find a storage site. So, even though you may have eaten only fat-free carbohydrates, you might as well have been eating pure lard.

Now, I want to be fair: not everyone has such a negative hormonal response to high-carbohydrate diets. There are people who can eat carbohydrates until the cows come home and never get fat. Why? It all depends on your genes.

Research conducted by Gerald Reaven at Stanford University in 1987 unraveled this genetic mystery. It turns out that people's genetic insulin responses to carbohydrates are diverse. In about 25 percent of a normal population, insulin response to carbohydrates is very blunted. When these lucky people eat excess carbohydrates, their insulin levels don't rapidly surge upward. They can consume large amounts of carbohydrates and not get hungry or fat. (These people often do very well on high-carbohydrate diets, so the dietary establishment elevates them to iconlike status to demonstrate the moral superiority of such a diet. Heck, these people just had a lucky draw in the genetic lottery.)

On the other hand, 25 percent of an otherwise normal population has an unlucky genetic draw that dictates an extremely elevated insulin response to carbohydrates. These people simply have to look at a carbohydrate and they begin gaining fat.

Between these two extremes lies the other 50 percent of the American population. These people respond normally to carbohydrates, which means that if they eat too much carbohydrate they'll have an elevated insulin response—not as elevated as the unluckiest 25 percent, but still elevated enough to do all the damage described above. These people will always fail on a high-carbohydrate diet. They're accused of being weak-willed gluttons who can't control themselves, when in fact they were just born with unfortunate genes.

This means that about one-quarter of the population who follow a high-carbohydrate diet will do reasonably well because they're blessed with genetic good fortune. These people can gorge themselves on carbohydrates and never get fat because their insulin levels are always low. The other 75 percent, however, will have an increasingly difficult time complying with such a diet. So, as I said, if you've failed on a high-carbohydrate diet, you're not at fault, your genes are. Well, you can't change your genes, but you sure can change your diet.

In later chapters, I'll spell out the rules for a diet that will allow you to escape from the hormonal consequences of carbohydrate hell and propel you into the Zone. For now, here's the bottom line: Eat small meals with the correct ratio of protein to carbohydrate. If you remember only that statement, you'll be positioning yourself for entry into the Zone.

In this chapter, I've talked mostly about the insulin-glucagon axis. But that axis is only one of hundreds of hormonal systems in the body. It's special because it controls glucose, the vital source of fuel for the brain. But perhaps even more important is its influence on the production of the vital superhormones called eicosanoids.

If insulin and glucagon are your portal to the Zone, eicosanoids *are* the Zone.

CHAPTER FOUR

EICOSANOIDS— THE SHORT COURSE

If hormones such as insulin and glucagon control blood sugar, what controls hormones? The answer: eicosanoids. In fact, eicosanoids (again, it's pronounced eye-KAH-sah-noids) are the body's superhormones. Mysterious and fleeting but all-powerful, eicosanoids are made by every living cell in the human body. They're the molecular glue that holds the human body together.

Not only do the eicosanoids control all of the body's hormonal systems, they control virtually every vital physiological function: the cardiovascular system, the immune system, the central nervous system, the reproductive system, and so on. When you get right down to it, eicosanoids are in charge of nothing less than keeping us alive and well. Without eicosanoids, life as we know it would be impossible.

The eicosanoid family includes a wide variety of superhormones with tongue-twisting names: prostaglandins, thromboxanes, leukotrienes, lipoxins, and hydroxylated fatty acids. I'll talk about these hormone groups and their effects on disease in more detail later on. For the moment just remember that *eicosanoids are the most powerful biological agents known to man. Control eicosanoids, and you'll open the door to the Zone.*

Yet, despite the crucial role eicosanoids play in maintaining life and health, they remain all but unknown. Your doctor has probably never heard of them. You can go to any medical school in the country, walk down the hallways, and ask any of the professors if they've ever heard of eicosanoids—after a blank stare, the answer is usually no.

This ignorance of eicosanoids in the medical community is amazing. The fact is that early discoveries in eicosanoid research won the 1982 Nobel Prize for Medicine, and the most powerful drugs in any medicine chest are designed to affect the levels of eicosanoids in the body.

The reason for this unfortunate ignorance is that eicosanoids are part of an axis of paracrine and autocrine hormones that are extremely complex, yet almost invisible. Their lifetimes are measured in seconds, they work at vanishingly low concentrations, and they don't use the bloodstream to reach their target tissues. In other words, like Greta Garbo, these hormones are rarely seen and therefore seldom understood.

Eicosanoids arise, do their jobs, then self-destruct, all in a flash. In many ways they're the biological equivalent of quarks in physics. Quarks are rarely observed. When they are it's usually only in gigantic particle accelerators, often after many years of experimental failure. Yet as difficult as quarks are to measure, any physicist will tell you that they are the foundation of all matter, and have been around since the beginning of time.

Eicosanoids aren't far behind. These superhormones have been around for more than five hundred million years—in fact, they were the first hormonal control system developed for living organisms. (Many of the eicosanoids that you and I produce are the same ones a sponge makes.) Even so, eicosanoids weren't discovered until 1936. Because they were isolated from the prostate gland, the first of the eicosanoids to be discovered were given the name *prostaglandins*.

At that point, it was thought that eicosanoids were simply another endocrine hormone system, secreted from the prostate gland to travel through the bloodstream to some unknown target cell. But their real role in the body could not be pinpointed. Eicosanoids lay all but dormant in the scientific literature for the next forty years.

It was only with the advent of more sophisticated instrumentation in the mid 1970s that eicosanoids could be studied for the first time. Since then there has been an explosion of knowledge (at least at the scientific research level), a continuing revelation as to how ubiquitous and powerful these hormones really are.

It turned out that prostaglandins represent only a few of the members in the larger family of eicosanoids. In the 1940s, scientists discovered another mysterious biochemical, which they first called *slow-reacting substance* (SRS). This discovery eventually led to an understanding of *leukotrienes*, another subclass of eicosanoids, which control, among other things, bronchial constriction and allergies.

Later in the 1970s came the discovery of *prostacyclins* and the *thromboxanes*—two of the key eicosanoids related to heart disease. In the 1980s still more groups of eicosanoids were uncovered, including *lipoxins* and *hydroxylated fatty acids*. These eicosanoids are important in controlling inflammatory responses and regulating the immune system.

All these eicosanoids operate at the level of the individual cell, and they have exceptionally diverse and powerful effects. In fact, the eicosanoids can be seen as the ultimate regulators of cellular function, turning cells on and off on a second-by-second basis—like fireflies lighting up a hot July evening.

"GOOD" AND "BAD" EICOSANOIDS

Like all hormones, eicosanoids operate as control systems. But, like insulin and glucagon, eicosanoids also have opposing actions. Since eicosanoids are the most powerful of all hormone systems, a balance of these opposing actions spells good health, and an imbalance spells disease. So, in effect, eicosanoids are your body's ultimate cellular check-and-balance system.

There's an even simpler way to put this: some eicosanoids are good, others are bad.

Of course, no natural substance is entirely good or entirely bad. As an example, take cholesterol. Doctors like to describe different varieties of cholesterol with the terms *good* (high-density lipoproteins, or HDL) and *bad* (low-density lipoproteins, or LDL). Well, as I said, there's no absolute good and there's no absolute bad in human physiology. Low-density lipoprotein (the carriers of bad cholesterol) are the molecular delivery trucks that transport the lipids, such as essential fatty acids and cholesterol, critical for cell growth. Without this bad cholesterol, you would die. It's when the *balance* of good and bad cholesterol becomes disturbed that the probability of cardiovascular trouble lurks ahead.

Another example, since we're talking about hormones, is insulin. As we saw in the previous chapter, too much insulin spells hypoglycemia (low blood sugar); too little can mean diabetes. The bottom line? Nature loves balance, and too much of a "good" thing (or too little of a "bad" thing) can in the end be bad.

The same is true of good and bad eicosanoids. But the physiologi-

**Eicosanoids Are
Controlled by Dietary Fat**

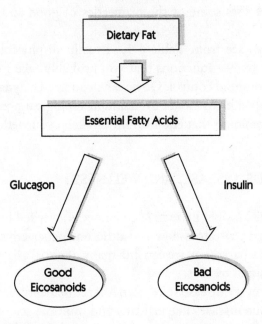

Figure 4-1

cal stakes are even higher because paracrine hormones like eicosanoids are much more powerful than endocrine hormones like insulin and glucagon.

Let's take platelet aggregation as an example. Platelet aggregation is simply a fancy term for the tendency of a type of blood cell known as platelets to join together to form clumps. Good eicosanoids prevent platelets from clumping (i.e., aggregating). Bad eicosanoids promote their clumping. When platelets clump together at the wrong time, you can develop a blood clot that may lead to a heart attack or stroke. But if you cut yourself, you want platelets to clump because that's what will eventually stop your bleeding. Too little of the bad eicosanoids, and you would bleed to death.

The same is true of blood pressure. Too many bad eicosanoids induce high blood pressure by causing constriction of the arteries (i.e., vasoconstriction). Too many good eicosanoids induce low blood pressure (i.e., vasodilation), which can lead to shock.

What's true for platelet aggregation and blood pressure is also true for pain, inflammation, the immune system, on and on: an imbalance of good and bad eicosanoids means disease.

Table 4-1 lists some of the properties of good and bad eicosanoids.

As you can see from Table 4-1, virtually all physiological functions in your body—functions that you probably take for granted—are under eicosanoid control. Obviously, you need a dynamic balance of good and bad eicosanoids to maintain biological equilibrium. In the end, maintaining that equilibrium can keep you well.

EICOSANOIDS, DISEASE, AND WELLNESS

When the 1982 Nobel Prize in Medicine was awarded for eicosanoid research, it gave rise to a new and different perspective on disease. Using this new paradigm, we can link many, if not all, disease states in a new and unified picture.

Virtually every disease state—whether it be heart disease, cancer, or autoimmune diseases like arthritis and multiple sclerosis—can be viewed at the molecular level as the body simply making more bad eicosanoids and fewer good ones. For some people that imbalance could mean heart disease, for others cancer, arthritis, or obesity.

If we turn that around, we'll see that redefining disease in terms of "good" and "bad" eicosanoids means that for the first time in medical history there is a simple but elegant molecular definition of wellness: the body making more "good" and fewer "bad" eicosanoids.

TABLE 4-1

Actions of Good and Bad Eicosanoids

GOOD EICOSANOIDS	BAD EICOSANOIDS
Inhibit platelet aggregation	Promote platelet aggregation
Promote vasodilation	Promote vasoconstriction
Inhibit cellular proliferation	Promote cellular proliferation
Stimulate immune response	Depress immune response
Anti-inflammatory	Pro-inflammatory
Decrease pain transmission	Increase pain transmission

WELLNESS VERSUS OPTIMAL HEALTH

Most of us define wellness as simply not being ill. The vast majority of people in America today may not be overtly ill, but they are definitely not feeling their best. *Optimal* health—the metabolic state in which the body and mind function at peak efficiency—goes beyond mere wellness. Optimal health is the state that all of us would like to reach.

Optimal health requires a balance of good and bad eicosanoids. As I said earlier, you must have some bad eicosanoids to survive, just as you have to have some bad cholesterol to survive. So, to achieve optimal health, the metabolic state you're after is the state in which the dynamic balance of good and bad eicosanoids is favorable. That is the molecular definition of the Zone.

What will the Zone, this state of optimal health, get you? Even if you're not ill, it will help prevent the likelihood of disease. Many chronic disease conditions such as obesity, heart disease, cancer, diabetes, depression, and alcoholism have a strong genetic linkage. The potential for their expression lies buried in your genetic code. In the Zone, you dramatically decrease the likelihood that those genes will be expressed. The further you are from the Zone, the more likely those genes will be expressed. More immediate, in the Zone you'll have greater access to stored body fat (instead of stored carbohydrate) for energy. You'll also benefit from greater mental concentration, which will not only help you be more productive, but will improve your physical performance as well.

Who could turn down the chance to reap these incredible benefits?

FOOD, EICOSANOIDS, AND THE ZONE

Whether you want to move from illness to wellness or beyond wellness to optimal health, your only pathway is through the Zone. How do you get to the Zone in the first place? It's amazingly simple: through the food you eat.

It's worth saying again: *If you follow a Zone-favorable diet, it will get you to the Zone and keep you there for the rest of your life.*

What is a Zone-favorable diet? It's a diet in which the balance of macronutrients—protein, carbohydrate, and fat—is tightly controlled: every meal, every snack, every day. What does macronutrient balance have to do with eicosanoids? First of all, dietary fat is the *only* source of the essential fatty acids that are the chemical building blocks for all eicosanoids. Meanwhile, the balance of protein and carbohydrate controls the insulin-glucagon axis, which in turn determines whether the eicosanoids your body makes are "good" or "bad." Pretty simple, actually.

Think of the body as a biological pinball machine. The pinballs (the essential fatty acids) are constantly being put into play by the plunger—the fat you eat at every meal. Whether the balls remain in play (making good eicosanoids) or end up in the well (making bad eicosanoids) depends upon how well you handle the flippers on the side of the machine. Those flippers are the combination of macronutrients in every meal and snack you eat.

Whether you know it or not, you play the eicosanoid game every four to six hours, every day of your life. The better you play the game, the better the results, and the more likely that you'll reach the Zone.

If you're consuming a diet that's too rich in carbohydrates—the same high-carbohydrate diet that is recommended for every cardiovascular patient, every athlete, and everyone else in America—then you're playing the game badly. Actually, you're doing everything in your power to make more bad eicosanoids. Why? Because you are causing an overproduction of insulin, and the resulting production of bad eicosanoids keeps your blood-sugar levels out of whack. This denies you access to your stored body fat, and ultimately leads to disease. Excess carbohydrates will drive you out of the Zone.

So, if you've been eating a high-carbohydrate diet, and you find yourself getting more fatigued, with less physical energy, and more and more body fat, now you know why. You've been playing the eicosanoid game poorly, and that poor play has short-circuited the basic control mechanisms—the eicosanoids—that have evolved over the last 500 million years to access your own stored body fat and maintain blood-sugar levels.

How do I know that playing the macronutrient game well—that

is, eating a Zone-favorable diet—will confer these benefits? I've tested it in heart patients, diabetics, overweight people, people with autoimmune diseases, even victims of HIV. But perhaps the most convincing tests were the ones I conducted in the best living laboratory of all: the bodies of world-class athletes.

CHAPTER FIVE

ELITE ATHLETES IN THE ZONE

Eight gold medals in swimming at Barcelona. Not a bad total for a major country, let alone a single American university. Add to that six consecutive NCAA swim championships in the past three years. What athletic factory has turned out such impressive results? It's no jock school. In fact, it's one of the toughest academic institutions in America: Stanford University.

The Stanford swimmers are among the hundreds of elite athletes I've worked with to help give them the advantage of competing in the Zone. The hormonal changes an elite athlete is trying to achieve by training are exactly the same changes a cardiovascular patient needs for wellness. In both cases, it's a question of making more good eicosanoids and fewer bad ones. In both cases, it's a question of being in the Zone.

You've learned that eating a high-carbohydrate diet is the surest way to stay out of the Zone. Yet high-carbohydrate diets are the foundation of current sports nutrition, especially for the top athletes in the world. The nutritionists are dead wrong.

Elite athletic performance is not determined on the day of competition, and it's certainly not dependent on some "energy" bar or drink. (By the way, most of the so-called "energy bars" on the market today are very high in carbohydrates and low in fat and protein. In macronutrient composition they're not much different from a conventional candy bar, except that candy bars taste better. The message: You can eat these "energy bars" all day long, and you'll never reach the Zone.)

Elite athletic performance is dependent on training and on the consistency of the diet for weeks or even months *prior* to the race or event. Nothing in the published scientific literature supports the current thinking that long-term consumption (longer than five days) of a high-carbohydrate diet improves athletic performance. A Zone-favorable diet, on the other hand, significantly enhances athletic performance in ways that can be scientifically measured. How do I know? I've spent the last four years examining that notion, and testing it on some of the world's best athletes. In essence, these athletes and their coaches have become a living laboratory.

My first opportunity to work with large groups of elite athletes in a quasi-clinical setting came in 1991, when former Los Angeles Raiders strength coach Marv Marinovich contacted me. Every summer Marv runs an ultra-intense training camp in southern California for college football players and professional basketball players. He had heard about the Zone through some of the work I was doing with Garrett Giemont, then the strength coach of the Los Angeles Rams, and with several of the Rams players.

When I first met Marv, he was twenty-five pounds overweight—even though he was one of the most knowledgeable trainers in America. Like almost everyone in the elite athletic establishment, Marv was an advocate of eating a high-carbohydrate diet. The first thing I did was encourage Marv to alter his diet to reach the Zone.

Marv was skeptical. How could all the experts in sports nutrition be wrong? At the same time, he knew of the great success that Garrett Giemont was having with the Los Angeles Rams players following a Zone-favorable diet. He decided to give it a try.

Two weeks later, Marv called me and said something remarkable was happening during his training. During one of his weight workouts, he said, "It was as if an anti-gravity breeze suddenly blew through the weight room." Now he was really interested in changing his entire nutritional approach to training.

So Marv was convinced, but his staff remained skeptical. Why did he want to change things? Hadn't his past dietary strategies always produced good results? Yes, but the possibility of getting even better results is what drives people like Marv, people on the cutting edge of top-level athletic training.

Marv asked if I would be interested in doing a pilot study with a larger group of nine elite athletes if he guaranteed that they would follow a Zone-favorable diet. My answer was an immediate yes.

This offer was so attractive because the type of study that Marv proposed would allow me to work with a larger group of trained athletes. The larger size of the group would provide the numbers to do statistical analysis. Now I could confirm scientifically that the results could be reproduced—just as they could be reproduced in the studies I had done with slightly overweight individuals. Statistics will tell you the probability that you can reproduce the results. If you have a probability factor of greater than 95 percent (a p factor of less than 0.05), then you're confident that if you repeat the same experiment 100 times, you'll get the same result 95 times. To do a proper statistical analysis, however, you need enough subjects who will follow directions for the course of the study. Marv's athletes fit the bill.

Also, this was an open pilot study to determine whether or not it was worth continuing any further research with elite athletes. If I couldn't get statistically significant performance improvement under these tightly controlled conditions, I never would.

So during the summer of 1991 we put nine of Marv's athletes (six top college football players and three professional basketball players) on a Zone-favorable diet for six weeks. Every meal was checked daily. If anyone brought a non-Zone-favorable meal to the camp, they got a warning from Marv. There was no second warning—the second time the athlete was out of the study and out of Marv's camp.

Okay, so Marv runs a tough camp. But this was the way he could ensure compliance with the diet.

Before the six-week period began, Marv measured the athletes' weight and percent of body fat, and calculated their lean body mass. At the same time, he tested their cardiovascular fitness, power (strength times speed), endurance, agility, and coordinated strength, using vertical jump (for lower body strength) and ability to throw a seven-pound ball (for upper body strength).

After six weeks on the Zone-favorable diet (and with intensive two-per-day training sessions), Marv measured and tested the athletes again. The results (given in Table 5-1) were astonishing, if not downright unbelievable. Their weight had increased by an average of more than eleven pounds, yet their amount of body fat had *dropped by five pounds*. This meant they had gained more than sixteen pounds of lean body muscle mass.

For such a relatively short time (six weeks), these changes in body composition were astonishing—especially since none of the athletes consumed more than 2,500 calories per day. But because they were continually in the Zone, the diet provided adequate amounts of pro-

TABLE 5-1

PARAMETER	% CHANGE	STATISTICAL SIGNIFICANCE (PROBABILITY FACTOR)
Body Composition		
Weight	+ 5%	$p < 0.005$
% Body fat	– 20%	$p < 0.005$
Lean body mass	+ 8%	$p < 0.005$
Performance		
Time to complete NFL agility run	– 2%	$p < 0.0005$
Cardiovascular fitness	+ 118%	$p < 0.0005$
Power	+ 30%	$p < 0.0005$
Last sprint time after 15 110-yd. sprints	– 7%	$p < 0.0005$
Overhead ball throw	+ 7%	$p < 0.0005$
Vertical jump	+ 10%	$p < 0.0005$

tein to repair and build new muscle tissue as well as maintain their existing lean body mass.

Changes in body composition, however, wasn't the important question I wanted to answer. I was more interested in performance. These athletes were chosen because they had already come off intensive spring conditioning programs and wanted to continue their conditioning program to be ready for September. As any top trainer will tell you, once you're at a peak level of conditioning, any further performance gains are usually very small. But without continuing workouts you can lose much of your performance edge. That loss of performance is called "detraining." For elite athletes detraining can occur within a matter of days. So the true test of Zone benefits would be if these athletes showed any significant performance *increases* during the six-week study period.

When Marv sent me the data for analysis, the results were so startling that I had to call him for confirmation. In fact, they were so startling to Marv that he was afraid to tell anyone. No exercise physiologist would have believed it. *Every one of the performance categories we tested improved, with a statistical significance of greater than 99.95 percent.* That meant if I repeated the same study 10,000 times, I would see performance improvement 9,995 times. Pretty good odds that the results were real, and not due to random chance.

And what were the results? First of all, the vertical jump, which indicates coordinated leg strength, improved by 10 percent. Here were athletes who had gained eleven extra pounds of weight, but were still able to increase their already impressive jumping ability by another three inches.

Next came endurance. Marv measured endurance by having the athletes run fifteen 110-yard sprints as fast as they could (with seventy-five seconds of rest between sprints), then comparing their times in the *last* sprint they ran. (I told you Marv is a tough taskmaster.) The results: the athletes were 7 percent faster in the last sprint than they had been at the beginning of the study period, *even though they were now on average eleven pounds heavier.* Yet, when they took the NFL agility test (remember Marv was the former strength coach of the Raiders), they were also significantly more agile.

Impressive as they were, these gains paled when compared to improvements in power and cardiovascular fitness. In football, strength is not as important as power. Power measures how fast you can move weight. Well, the athletes showed an average power improvement of 30 percent. And their cardiovascular fitness—perhaps the most important category in terms of overall health—increased by an amazing 118 percent.

Marv's summary of the study: "Unbelievable."

Today every athlete Marv trains has to make a commitment to eat a Zone-favorable diet. Oh, by the way—Marv himself lost twenty pounds, and now is stronger and has better endurance than he had when he played linebacker for the Raiders some twenty-five years ago.

With the completion of Marv's study, I knew that elite athletes could expect significant performance gains if they trained in the Zone. But what about elite athletes in free living conditions, when they didn't have Marv inspecting their food choices? After all, Marv ran his camp as if it were a metabolic ward in a hospital.

Here's where I got my second break. Through a mutual friend, I had an opportunity to meet Richard Quick and Skip Kenney, coaches of the men's and women's swim teams at Stanford University. Richard and Skip are probably the top two swim coaches in the country, if not the world. Like Marv, they're at the cutting edge of athletic training, and looking for every trick in the book to improve their athletes' performance.

And like Marv, Richard and Skip were skeptical. So the first thing I suggested to Richard and Skip was that they try the program themselves. I figured I would wait for about two weeks, as I had for Marv and Garrett Giemont.

After two weeks, each coach called me independently and said they could not believe the difference. Their own results, coupled with the data accumulated from Marv's athletes, convinced them that the Zone could be the last spoke in the wheel to maximize performance for elite swimmers at a world-class level. With the 1992 Olympics coming up, they asked if I would work with their teams during the upcoming year. What another great opportunity!

So, in effect, the Stanford pool became an ongoing laboratory, where we could compare the effects of a Zone-favorable diet on a group of swimmers with those of other elite swimmers who followed the standard high-carbohydrate diets recommended by the experts.

Nineteen ninety-two was an important year, both for the team and for the individual athletes. For the past two years, the University of Texas swimmers (both men and women) had consistently beaten Stanford badly in the NCAA swimming championships. (At the time, the University of Texas was considered to have the top swimming program in the country.) As individuals, the Stanford athletes were also trying to make the United States team that would compete at the 1992 Olympics in Barcelona. The challenge was formidable, made even more difficult by a brutal schedule—the Olympic trials were held in March, and the NCAA championships only a few weeks later.

Let's be frank: at first, not all kids on the Stanford teams bought into the Zone program. After all, they'd been eating carbohydrates until their eyes bulged out, and had done fine. Why change anything now? But those Stanford swimmers who did follow the diet with the same degree of compliance that Marv's athletes had shown dramatically altered their athletic futures.

At the Olympic trials in Indianapolis, six of the Stanford swimmers qualified for the team. Not surprisingly (to me, at least), these were the swimmers who followed a Zone-favorable diet most faithfully. Two weeks later, the Stanford women overcame a home-pool advantage—the NCAA championships were held on the University of Texas campus in Austin—and finally wrested the NCAA title from Texas, by a score of 735 to 651. The following week, the Stanford men duplicated the triumph, breaking Texas's four-year stranglehold on the men's title.

As sweet as these victories were, the parade of Stanford titles was just beginning. At the Olympics in Barcelona that summer, Stanford swimmers won eight gold medals—three individual events and as members of two relay teams. This was nearly one-third of the total gold medal wins by American swimmers, and it was only one medal less than the total number won by the entire German team, which had dominated Olympic swimming since 1976. In the course of that breakthrough year, the Stanford swimmers set two new world records, and obliterated a number of American and collegiate records.

"We knew we had the potential to have a great year in 1992," Coach Skip Kenney said later, "but what the teams actually accomplished was way beyond anything we might have expected."

Since then, Stanford swim teams—both men's and women's—have won their respective NCAA titles every year (1992, 1993, and 1994), dominating the championships and setting new competitive standards. Meanwhile, individual Stanford swimmers have also achieved breakthrough performances.

For example, a Zone-favorable diet helped former Stanford star Angie Wester-Krieg become the oldest woman, at twenty-eight, ever to make an American Olympic swim team. The same diet helped Pablo Morales come back from three years on the sidelines to win two Olympic gold medals at the unheard-of age of twenty-seven.

Among the individual Stanford swimmers, though, there's no better example than Jenny Thompson. As a high school competitor, Jenny had been one of the top freestyle swimmers in the country. But in her senior year in high school her performances hit a plateau. Since she was already signed to swim for Stanford after graduation, Coach Quick asked me to talk to her before she traveled to Stanford in September.

At the trials in Indianapolis, Jenny proved the point. She swam the 100-meter freestyle in 54.48 seconds, beating her previous personal best by almost a full second, and breaking a world record that had stood for six years. (If you're familiar with swimming, you know that world records rarely last six months, but this one had been set by an East German swimmer on anabolic steroids; thus its unusual longevity.) Weeks later, at the NCAA championships in Austin, Jenny smashed the American record in the 100-yard freestyle. And in the Barcelona Olympics that summer, she took a silver medal in the 100-meter freestyle and two gold medals as anchor in the 400-meter medley and 400-meter freestyle relays.

"Some people were saying that Jenny must have been doing something illegal to swim the way she did," Coach Quick told *Swimming World* in a 1993 article. "They thought there was no way she could have gone as fast as she did without drugs.

"But I can absolutely guarantee that wasn't the case. It was the dietary program outlined by Dr. Sears."

Marv Marinovich's athletes and the Stanford swimmers were not the only world-class athletes to reap the rewards of a Zone-favorable diet. Over the past five years, the program has helped hundreds of elite athletes achieve a wide variety of personal goals. Eating a Zone-favorable diet helped NBA star James Donaldson prolong his professional career. "At thirty-five," he says, "I was outrunning and outlasting players in their twenties." Now at age 39, he is the starting center for the Utah Jazz. It helped downhill ski racer Lisa Feinberg win the U.S. Masters championship. It helped Dutch sprinter Miguel Jannsen break the Netherlands national record in the 200-meter sprint, even though he was running against an 8-mph head wind. It helped Masters swimmer Phil Whitten break four world age-group records, and it helped triathlete Laura Lowe win the 1994 Maui Ironman. And my Zone-favorable diet also helped Dave Scott—known as the godfather of triathletes—finish second in the 1994 Gatorade Ironman Triathlon—at the age of forty, and after a layoff of five years.

What explains these remarkable results? What did a Zone-favorable diet do for these athletes that allowed them to boost their performance levels so dramatically? To answer these questions, we have to go inside the athletes' bodies and see what's really going on when they're putting themselves to the ultimate physical tests.

All athletic performance at the elite level is ultimately dependent on adaptation to continued training. At the molecular level, this adaptation requires the complex orchestration of various hormonal systems that enables an athlete to perform at higher work loads.

Understanding how training and diet affect these hormonal systems is the real key to achieving maximum athletic performance. Once you understand the adverse hormonal effects that result from eating a high-carbohydrate diet, it should become obvious why it's hormonally impossible for a high-carbohydrate diet to generate maximum performance. To put it simply, elite athletes who eat a high-carbohydrate diet will never consistently reach the Zone, where true maximal potential is realized.

Well, you might ask, if that's true, how are elite athletes who are on high-carb diets still managing to break records? Of course, top athletes can perform well outside the Zone because of their natural abilities and their disciplined training. But inside the Zone they can perform even better.

Staying in the Zone gives these athletes a huge advantage over the athletes who are still buying into the high-carbohydrate myth. You see, the typical athlete's diet is basically the same diet that is making America fat. To make matters worse, the carbohydrates these athletes eat come primarily from "unfavorable" high-glycemic sources like pasta. (Usually, when athletes talk about "carbo loading" the day before a competition, they means stuffing themselves with enormous mounds of pasta.)

What are the hormonal consequences? Athletes on high-carbohydrate diets are forcing their bodies to produce too much insulin, which in turn keeps their cells churning out "bad" eicosanoids. This unfortunate combination reduces oxygen transfer to the muscle cells, thus reducing endurance and overall physical performance. At the same time, this ongoing hyperinsulinemia spells constant hunger, setting up a vicious circle if the athlete uses carbohydrates to appease that hunger.

Overproduction of insulin and "bad" eicosanoids also denies the athlete access to stored body fat, so that most of the energy he or she needs has to come from a very limited source: carbohydrates. Equally important, a high-carbohydrate diet means increased muscle fatigue and decreased mental alertness.

As a matter of fact, the newest scientific studies are now beginning to show that at least as far as elite athletes are concerned, the high-carbohydrate diet may be highly overrated. One of those studies, conducted in 1990 by a team of researchers at Ohio State University, compared the effects of two different diets on the training intensity of a group of college swimmers. One of the diets derived about 40 percent of total calories from carbohydrates, the other 80 percent.

After the nine-day test period was over, the researchers put the swimmers in the pool and timed them for various distances. The results? The times of the swimmers on the high-carbohydrate diets were no better than those on the more moderate diet. For swim-training intensity, the scientists concluded, "an 80 percent carbohydrate diet provides no advantage."

When this same team of Ohio State scientists did a similar study in 1993, this one involving runners and cyclists, they came to the same conclusion: high-carbohydrate diets generated no performance enhancement.

To exercise physiologists, these studies must have come as bad news. But another controlled study, this one published in 1994 by David Pendergast and his colleagues at the Sports Medicine Institute of the State University of New York at Buffalo, must have been downright embarrassing in terms of its implications for elite athletes and high-carbohydrate diets.

The SUNY study compared the effects of a high-fat versus a high-carbohydrate diet on the endurance of six elite distance runners. In both diets the amounts of protein remained constant. But the high-fat diet provided more than 150 grams of fat per day. (This is a massive amount of fat, far more than ever recommended on a Zone-favorable diet.)

In this study, the runners were treated like Marv Marinovich's athletes. Each meal was planned for the athletes, and every meal had to be recorded for the researchers by the athletes. (In essence, these elite athletes were treated like lab rats.) Each runner tried each diet for seven days, and at the end of the seventh day, each took an endurance test, running on a treadmill until he reached exhaustion.

The results? The runners on the high-fat diet—that is, the diet with the lowest amount of carbohydrate—had the best endurance time. When the runners were switched to a high-carbohydrate diet, with a much lower protein-to-carbohydrate ratio, their endurance dropped by 20 percent, and their maximal oxygen consumption was 10 percent lower. A dramatic decrease in performance in only seven days. The bottom line: high-carbohydrate diets actually *limited* the performance of these highly trained endurance athletes.

Of course, this research just confirms my earlier work with Marv Marinovich's athletes and the Stanford swimmers. It may also explain why there are no ranked Americans in the marathon or in long-distance swimming, since endurance athletes in this country treat carbohydrates as if they were manna from heaven, and in the process reduce potential endurance performance.

But that's not the end of it. In studies at the University of Texas, it's been shown that meals containing both protein and carbohydrate are superior to carbohydrate alone in replacing muscle glycogen and promoting the release of growth hormone after intensive exercise. Both of these biochemical events are critical to improve recovery times after intensive workouts. That's just what the Stanford swimmers do when they eat a Zone-favorable snack after each practice.

Of course, all these studies were short-term—none lasted longer than nine days. But what happens after nine weeks, or nine months? One possible inference can be made by comparing the Stanford swimmers to the University of Texas swimmers since 1992. After all, before 1992 the University of Texas had been the dominant swim team in both men's and women's swimming. And the NCAA championships at the end of the season provide an ideal comparison platform, since everything is on the line at the same time and in the same pool.

Although far from a scientific study, the results of the 1992 championships are very interesting. Compared to previous years, the difference in the number of points scored by Stanford and Texas teams, both men and women, represented a complete reversal. Those results are shown in Figure 5-1. What caused that reversal? The Stanford coaches believe it was the introduction of a Zone-favorable diet. I agree.

At the elite level, all athletes are genetically gifted. They all have excellent training discipline, and they all have great coaches. The difference between first and fifth place is exceedingly small. As a result, diet can play a major role in determining who finishes first and who finishes fifth. But diet works in both directions. As all these studies have shown, a high-carbohydrate diet is likely to reduce the athlete's capability to achieve maximum performance.

If an athlete hopes to perform at his or her best, he or she must understand how to use diet to both train and compete in the Zone. A Zone-favorable diet, with its appropriate balance of eicosanoids, provides the athlete with a number of immediate benefits. Calorie consumption is usually cut by as much as 50 percent, because the athlete is accessing stored body fat as a primary source of energy, instead of having to eat extra food—especially energy-poor carbohydrates—to get the necessary energy.

Yet even though caloric intake is reduced in a Zone-favorable diet, constant hunger, especially those cravings for carbohydrates, is eliminated because blood-sugar levels are maintained at a more or

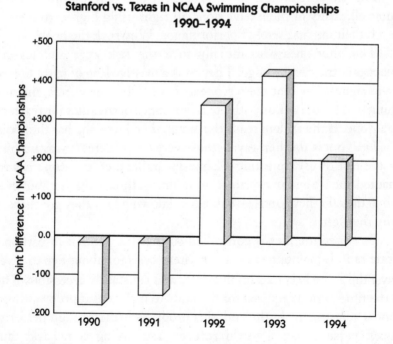

Stanford vs. Texas in NCAA Swimming Championships
1990–1994

Figure 5-1

less constant level for four to six hours—the amount of time between Zone-favorable meals.

The hormonal benefits generated by a Zone-favorable diet produce unprecedented gains in athletic performance. In the Zone, fatty acids are released from adipose tissue at a faster rate, meaning increased muscular endurance because muscle glycogen is conserved. Stored fat is better utilized, both during training and at rest, and this provides the desirable fat loss that almost all athletes seek. Oxygen transfer is increased and muscle fatigue minimized. And stable blood-sugar levels provide increased mental alertness—indispensable if an athlete expects to achieve maximum performance.

If all this is true—and both my own work and the most recent studies of other researchers strongly suggest that it is—why haven't the sports nutrition experts acknowledged the results? Because it takes courage to change the dietary "wisdom," especially if there's an elaborate existing establishment to explain why long-term adherence to high-carbohydrate diets improves performance—even if the data doesn't support the concept.

For the elite athlete or the coach, it takes even more courage. After all, many of them have done all right using high-carb diets to reach their current level of performance. Why rock the boat?

The only ones who initially took the risk were athletes and coaches at the cutting edge. They took a massive leap of faith, hoping I was right. Now that these pioneers have tested the waters, the only thing that holds back any athlete is ignorance of the rules for reaching the Zone. If the athlete reads this book, then he or she has the tools.

Let's put it another way: because very few athletes (to say nothing of the rest of us) are eating a Zone-favorable diet, the Zone has remained elusive and mysterious. Sometimes athletes reach it, but even when they do they soon leave it, never knowing how they got there or why they left.

But once the diet is controlled so that the protein-to-carbohydrate ratio is maintained on a consistent basis for about five to seven days, the Zone becomes immediately and constantly accessible. This is the time period required for the body to make the appropriate hormonal adjustment. In the end, this produces breakthrough performances, personal bests, world records, astounding comebacks, and roomfuls of championship trophies.

Once elite athletes, their coaches, and their nutritionists come to this realization, athletic performances will jump to new levels, with records falling like tin soldiers. It's just a matter of time. Until then, the Stanford coaches and the other elite athletes I've worked with are hoping their competitors continue their pasta-loading ways.

CHAPTER SIX

EXERCISE IN THE ZONE

We know why elite athletes exercise—it's their job. But what about the rest of us? Why do most people exercise? To lose weight and, they hope, change the way they look in a swimsuit. But the sad truth is that the health-club industry is built on ninety-day wonders: people who join a club to get in shape—that is, to lose excess body fat. These instant fitness buffs buy Spandex outfits, train religiously, and sweat profusely. Ninety days later, when they haven't changed their body shape one iota, they quit.

Or if they don't join a health club, they buy an expensive piece of home exercise equipment. Ninety days later, that gleaming home gym is nothing but a high-priced clothes rack.

It's ironic that the fattest country in the world has the most health clubs and the greatest variety of home exercise equipment on the face of the earth. Americans join more health clubs than anyone else in the world. What's going on here? Has exercising in health clubs made America fat? Or is it that all this formal exercise simply can't overcome the hormonal consequences of a high-carbohydrate diet?

There's no doubt that exercise should be a vital part of any personal total health program, not only because of its well-known "sweat benefits"—improved weight control, improved cardiovascular fitness, and improved strength—but also because of the sense of well-being that comes from even mild exertion. But what's the real biological source of these benefits? They're simply a consequence of the hormonal changes that various types of exercise induce.

Ask any trainer about the hormonal effects of exercise, and most of them will look at you as if you just arrived from Mars. Ask nutritionists (or other nutrition experts—like your next-door neighbor) about the hormonal effects of food, and they'll give you the same blank look.

Well, I hope that by now I've persuaded you to think of food as a modulator of hormones. And you should think of exercise in the same way. When you think hormonally, you understand that exercise and food go hand in glove; and you want to ensure that the hormonal benefits of exercise are being enhanced, not destroyed, by the hormonal effects of the food you eat.

Yes, food is still the primary pathway to the Zone, but exercise can help widen that path and make it easier to stay in the Zone on a long-term basis. (Remember, you can't exercise all day long, but you probably eat several times every day.) This simply means that all the exercise in the world may never get you to the Zone if you're following the wrong diet.

What's the wrong diet? The standard high-carbohydrate diet. To understand why this is true, you have to understand the relationships between food, exercise, and energy. And you have to understand what the hormonal effects of exercise actually are.

BURNING CALORIES VERSUS BURNING FAT

Most people think that the goal of exercise is to burn calories. In fact, you'll replace most of the calories you burn in most forms of aerobic exercise just by eating one or two bran muffins. At the same time, any hormonal benefits of exercise will disappear, as the two muffins you eat will immediately send you out of the Zone.

Fat, not carbohydrate, is the primary source of energy for your muscles. Not only is fat a more efficient raw-material source for energy generation—fat actually supplies more than twice the energy of carbohydrates—it is also far more plentiful. A world-class marathon runner, for example, will have twenty times more energy stored as fat than as carbohydrates in his or her body.

Sound ridiculous? Let's look at the math. Completing a typical marathon will require about 2,000 calories of energy. That also happens to be the maximum amount of carbohydrate a marathoner can store in the muscles and liver: about 2,000 calories. If the marathon runner uses only his stored carbohydrates, he or she may not have enough energy to complete the race.

On the other hand, if the same 150-pound marathoner has 10 percent body fat, this translates into 15 pounds of total fat. About 3 pounds of that total fat is not accessible for energy because it's in places like the brain. This leaves about 12 pounds of fat for possible energy use.

Since there are 3,500 calories per pound of fat, this amount of accessible fat potentially provides the runner with 42,000 calories of energy—more than twenty times the energy available from stored carbohydrates. If he or she can use his own stored fat, the runner actually has enough energy to run more than twenty marathons! So which fuel should he or she want to use? The answer should be obvious: fat.

Of course, few of us actually run marathons. So let's take a look at what's happening at the other end of the energy spectrum. Most of the energy the body needs is used simply to keep warm. To keep the furnace stoked, we all carry with us two sources of energy: stored body fat and stored carbohydrate.

But the primary fuel used to keep the body warm is fat. In fact, when you're sitting in a chair, fat provides about 70 percent of the calories needed to keep the body warm and functioning. As long as you stay in the chair (or in any sedentary position), the flow of fat from the storage depot (the adipose tissue) along the superhighway (the bloodstream) to the factory (the muscles) is easily maintained.

So even when you're just sitting in front of a TV set, you're still burning fat—just not very much of it. Nonetheless your heart is still pumping at some level. Let's assume you are 50 years old, and you have a resting heart rate of 72. Your maximum heart rate (using the standard formula of 220 minus your age) would be about 170 beats per minute. Watching TV requires a heart rate of 72 beats a minute. If I divide 72 by 170, that tells me you require 42 percent of your maximum heart rate simply to watch TV. You probably didn't think you were working so hard when you were channel-surfing.

Now let's suppose you want to go to the refrigerator for a snack. That's going to require a little more energy, so your heart rate speeds up slightly because you're moving. But you're still burning fat, just as you did when you were sitting in your TV chair.

Now let's move up a notch. There will be some point at which you'll be doing something at least a little more strenuous than going to the refrigerator and back to the TV. Whatever that activity might be, it will increase the demands for muscle contraction. At that point you have to burn still more of your body's fuel (either stored fat or stored carbohydrate) to generate energy so that your muscles can contract for a more extended period of time. This is called exercise.

When you exercise, you begin to place greater work demands on the body. So you have to get more fat from the storage depot to the factory—the muscles. What's the controlling factor in the release of fat from your storage depot? You guessed it: it's the balance of eicosanoids. When you're in the Zone, which means that your body is making more good eicosanoids and fewer bad ones, the fat you require to meet your energy needs can be released faster. As you move out of the Zone, the fat release drops to a trickle. The factories will then reluctantly switch to an inferior, lower-octane fuel: carbohydrate.

So no matter what your level of exercise—whether you're just watching TV or whether you're grinding your way through a marathon—if you're out of the Zone, you're burning stored carbohydrate instead of stored body fat.

Here's how the process works in a little more detail. Muscle contractions require a unique chemical energy source called *adenosine triphosphate* (ATP). This energy source is rapidly used up with each muscle contraction and has to be replaced if you want more muscle contractions.

Making more of this energy source requires a lot of raw materials. So the workers (enzymes) in the factories use the best available raw materials (fat or carbohydrate). They'd rather have fat, because it's a more efficient energy source and the body has a lot of it. (Carbohydrate is less efficient and you can't store much of it.) But if they can't get the fat they prefer, the enzymes switch to carbohydrate.

What does this mean to the average person who wants to exercise simply to lose excess body fat? It means understanding what really goes on when you exercise, both aerobically and anaerobically. As I said, it means understanding the hormonal effects of exercise.

AEROBIC EXERCISE

Aerobic is a space-age word, but don't let that fool you: aerobic exercise simply means exercising in the presence of oxygen. If you only want to burn excess body fat for energy—that is, if you're less concerned with building strength or lean body mass—then aerobic exercise is for you.

The usual prescription for aerobic exercise is to do some kind of activity that raises your heart rate to some percentage of its maximum. Your maximum heart rate depends on your age, and decreases as you get older. As I stated earlier, a good approximation of your maximum heart rate is 220 minus your age.

If you've ever been to a health club, the trim and perky instructor probably told you that the only way to burn fat is to maintain the intensity of your aerobic exercise at 70 percent of your maximum heart rate and keep it there for twenty minutes or more. In a way, this advice is correct (more about that in a moment), but it's too simplistic. It overlooks the way your body chooses its exercise fuel.

Obviously, you want to burn more fat than carbohydrate when you exercise. But if you begin exercising too hard, the demand on getting the fat from where it's located (the adipose tissue) to where you make energy (the muscles) is often the limiting step. If the muscles can't get enough fat, they switch over to using the stored carbohydrate that sits within the muscle. If you stick to the standard health-club prescription for exercise intensity, you're making energy for the muscles, but you're actually using less stored fat.

How to get around this dilemma? One way is to exercise for longer periods of time, and at a lower maximum heart rate, than recommended by the aerobic instructors at the local gym. (Remember that just sitting in your chair your heart is beating at 42 percent of its maximum rate.)

What's the best exercise to achieve this? It's called walking. Have you ever wondered why Europeans aren't fat? They don't go to aerobic classes, they just walk a lot.

The latest research indicates that the maximum benefits for increased longevity occur after you expend more than 2,000 calories per week on exercise. Above that level, there's no further benefit. Well, it's very easy to achieve that level of total calorie expenditure by walking every day. Walking uses slightly more than 300 calories per hour. If you walk six hours per week—less than an hour per day—you'll burn all the calories you need to get the vital "sweat benefits," thus reducing your overall risk of dying before your time.

Higher-intensity exercises, like jogging, burn about twice as many calories per hour as walking does. So if you don't want to spend six hours per week walking, plan to spend three hours per week jogging. Remember, that's three *hours* a week—not the thirty minutes three times a week that's usually recommended. An hour and a half a week of jogging simply won't work as well as six hours of walking.

Consider this: the average American spends 3 hours per day in front of a TV—that's 21 hours a week. If that average American is in the Zone, he or she will burn more body fat during those 21 hours than in 1 1/2 hours of jogging. (Of course, if he or she isn't in the Zone, all bets are off.)

So if it's true that you can burn body fat simply by walking—or even by watching TV—why listen to that aerobics instructor who tells you that the only way to burn off that excess body fat is to do aerobic exercise at high intensities? Well, it turns out that the aerobics instructors are right, but for the wrong reasons.

The real key—and few aerobics instructors know this—is that the higher the intensity of exercise, the more hormonal responses are affected. Specifically, higher-intensity aerobic exercise reduces insulin levels, and increases levels of glucagon. Sound familiar? It should, because that's exactly what a Zone-favorable diet does.

It's the same story: if you decrease insulin, you begin to make more good eicosanoids and fewer bad ones. This favorable balance of eicosanoids means you're releasing more stored body fat from the adipose tissue. So when you're in the Zone, you've set the conditions for maximal fat release. And you're burning fat, not carbohydrates. That's why you want high-intensity aerobic exercise.

If burning fat were the only hormonal benefit of high-intensity aerobic exercise, that would still be enough to make it healthy and wise. But there's another hormonal reward that comes from exercising in the Zone: the good eicosanoids you generate dilate your blood vessels, increasing the transfer of oxygen from the blood to the muscles. Once your body can no longer transfer sufficient oxygen to the muscles, it becomes impossible to use fat for energy. In the Zone (where oxygen transfer is increased) you can stay in aerobic metabolism for longer periods of time even during increased exercise demands.

As you exercise with higher levels of intensity, you begin to create the hormonal changes that are the real fruits of exercise—just as hormonal changes are the real power of nutrition.

The intensity range of exercise that induces an improved balance of eicosanoids is between 60 and 80 percent of your maximum heart rate. There are many forms of exercise that can generate that level of intensity: jogging, running, swimming, or skipping rope. Unfortunately, these tend to be boring because you have to do them continuously—without stopping for breaks—to have a positive hormonal effect.

Playing sports like racquetball, tennis, or basketball is a lot more fun, but the action is not continuous, so there are fewer hormonal benefits. Most of the quick bursts of action in these sports force you over the intensity limit. Beyond that intensity limit, the rate of oxygen transfer to the muscle cells is no longer great enough to maintain aerobic metabolism. At that point your muscle cells must switch to anaerobic metabolism (energy conversion in the absence of oxygen), where it's impossible to use fat to make more energy.

So to get the maximum hormonal benefits from aerobic exercise, activities like jogging, swimming, rowing, and skipping rope are probably the best. If you find those activities boring, wear a Walkman—there are even water-resistant models for swimming. Or, while you exercise, use that time to meditate, plan your investment strategies, calculate your next move at work—or even make up the guest list for your next Zone-favorable dinner party.

ANAEROBIC EXERCISE

From a hormonal point of view, at first glance anaerobic exercise (weight lifting, resistance training, or interval training [wind sprints] in running and swimming) looks like a bad bet. First of all, because oxygen transfer is very limited under anaerobic conditions, the muscles can no longer make energy from fat. They're forced to use stored carbohydrate. So much for burning fat—or so it seems.

Now for more apparently bad news. The efficiency of energy generation in anaerobic exercise falls to about 5 percent of what it was under conditions of aerobic metabolism. So it seems that anaerobic exercise isn't giving you very much bang for the buck in terms of burning fat for energy, and it's rapidly depleting a very limited energy source (stored carbohydrate) at the same time.

If all this is true—especially if anaerobic exercise won't burn fat—then why would anybody in their right mind want to exercise that way? After all, even if running is boring, it sure is a lot more fun than wind sprints or lifting weights. Well, for most people the goal of anaerobic exercise is simply to build muscle. That's because current mythology has it that the only way to burn fat is through aerobic exercise.

Guess what? Once again the current "wisdom" is wrong. Although anaerobic exercise doesn't access fat directly, it still has a powerful indirect effect on the fat-burning process.

What is that effect? If the intensity of the anaerobic workout is high enough, it causes the body to release human growth hormone. This exceptionally potent hormone has a number of important jobs in the body, one of which is to repair the microdamage done to muscle tissue during anaerobic exercise. It takes a lot of energy to do the repair job, and that energy comes from your stored body fat.

This means that, in effect, *human growth hormone is the most powerful fat-burning hormone in the body.* So release of human growth hormone from the pituitary gland is the crucial hormonal change that occurs with anaerobic exercise. That hormonal change gives you two crucial sweat benefits: it burns fat, and it allows you to build new muscle at the same time. (And what controls the release of human growth hormone from the pituitary gland? Good eicosanoids.)

A number of scientific studies, including a famous one by Daniel Rudman and his colleagues at the Medical College of Wisconsin in Milwaukee, have shown that injections of human growth hormone are something like an elixir of youth—even for people over sixty-five. In the Rudman study, reported in the *New England Journal of Medicine* in 1991, older men who were injected with human growth hormone for six months lost body fat and gained lean body mass. In fact, the researchers stated that in terms of body composition it was as if the old men were now fifteen years younger.

Another study, this one using trained weight lifters, was conducted at the University of New Mexico Medical School in 1988. Half the weight lifters got injections of growth hormone during their six weeks of training, while the other half received injections of saline solution. At the end of six weeks, those who got the growth-hormone injections (providing more than 50% greater amounts than normal blood levels) had lost four times more body fat and gained four times more lean body mass than those who got the placebo injections. (Incidentally, these were the same kinds of body-composition changes achieved in Marv Marinovich's athletes when they were following a Zone-favorable diet. But the changes on the Zone-favorable diet were twice as great as those in the growth-hormone study.)

The results of these studies are eye-opening, because they highlight the power of human growth hormone. But injections of the hormone are a difficult and dangerous way to trim fat and build muscle. First of all, human growth hormone is FDA approved only for the treatment of unusually small children. Any other use is illegal. Secondly, injecting this powerful hormone has some potent adverse side effects, including shutting down the body's natural release of the hormone, and increasing the risk of developing diabetes.

Luckily, you don't have to inject growth hormone to burn fat and build muscle. All you have to do is train anaerobically. But you do have to understand that you only begin to exercise anaerobically when you are at levels in excess of 90 percent of your maximum heart rate. This is pretty hard work. It's also why world-class sprinters and swimmers are heavily muscled and at the same time very lean—they train anaerobically.

By the way, there is one other time that growth hormone is released, and it has nothing to do with training. It's released during sleep; actually during stage 3 and 4 just prior to REM (Rapid Eye Movement) sleep. This is the time in which your body repairs itself for the next day of operation. The better the quality of your sleep, the more growth hormone will be released during your sleep.

So how do you maximize growth-hormone release during sleep? Eat a Zone-favorable snack before you retire. That snack will set in motion the hormonal foundation to allow maximum secretion of growth hormone. On the other hand, if you eat a carbohydrate-rich snack before you go to bed, you've done everything in your power to inhibit growth hormone release. Why? Because you've raised insulin levels, and insulin retards the secretion of growth hormone from the pituitary gland.

That is why one consequence of being out of the Zone is the "sleep paradox": you sleep longer, but still find yourself very groggy upon waking. On the other hand, in the Zone the sleep paradox is turned on its head: you need less sleep, but you're more alert when you wake up. So if you want to enjoy the hormonal benefits of anaerobic exercise while you sleep, stay in the Zone.

EXERCISE IN THE ZONE

Why do you want to exercise when you're in the Zone? Because in the Zone all of the beneficial hormonal changes caused by exercise (both aerobic and anaerobic) are accelerated. But if you're training outside the Zone, many of the hormonal benefits of exercise are negated.

For example: let's say that you're eating a high-carbohydrate meal or snack—perhaps one of those sports "energy" bars, which are loaded with carbohydrates—right after you exercise. Those carbohydrates will drive you right out of the Zone. They'll raise your insulin levels, and, since insulin is a powerful inhibitor of human growth hormone, the release of human growth hormone that you expected from exercise will be muted.

Being out of the Zone means you're making too much insulin and not enough good eicosanoids. This means your anaerobic exercise program is less likely to do what it's intended to do: build muscle and trim fat.

In aerobic exercise the same sad tale is true. Remember that high levels of insulin generated by too much carbohydrate drive you out of the Zone by decreasing the production of good eicosanoids and increasing the production of bad ones. As your eicosanoid balance changes for the worse, you can't access body fat as effectively during exercise, and the oxygen transfer rate is dramatically reduced. The end result: you're burning more stored carbohydrate and less stored body fat. So your aerobic exercise program isn't making you any leaner—especially when you consider the amount of time you're spending at the gym.

The bottom line: if you want to generate the maximum hormonal benefits from exercise, aerobic or anaerobic or both, you need to be in the Zone—before you exercise, while you exercise, and right after you exercise. This is true whether you're a marathon runner, a weight lifter, a jogger, or a three-times-a-week aerobic dancer.

How do you accomplish this? Eat a Zone-favorable snack thirty minutes before exercising. The hormonal changes caused by a Zone-favorable snack (see Appendix D) will allow you to access stored body fat more effectively during your exercise. In other words, you'll be burning fat faster. Then, right after you finish exercising, eat another Zone-favorable snack.

Remember: no matter how modest or lofty your exercise goals, a high-carbohydrate diet may keep you from achieving them. If you're eating too much carbohydrate, you can expect the following, even if you're on a judicious program of aerobic exercise: constant hunger, decreased mental alertness, difficulty in losing body fat (if not out-right fat gain), decreased oxygen transfer to the muscle cells, and decreased endurance. *All of these are consequences of being out of the Zone.*

If you want the maximum hormonal rewards from exercise, staying in the Zone is the key. How do you get the hormonal benefits of exercise twenty-four hours a day? Make every meal a Zone-favorable meal.

Think of being in the Zone as dietary cross-training. Whether you're running, swimming, pumping iron, or doing any other form of ongoing exercise, this dietary cross-training—the combination of a Zone-favorable diet with a continuing exercise program—will soon mean a newer, stronger, and better you.

CHAPTER SEVEN

BOUNDARIES OF THE ZONE

How do you maintain a favorable balance of eicosanoids? How do you get to the Zone? Those two questions are actually one and the same, and they have the same answer: through the Zone-favorable dietary technology I've developed. Like any other technology, a dietary technology has rules. A dietary technology has defined boundaries, and it works on simple scientific principles.

In this chapter, I'd like to show you the primary rule for keeping your eicosanoids in healthy balance. Although there are other signposts on the pathway to the Zone, you can shorten the path if you follow my one cardinal rule.

What is that rule? Maintain a beneficial ratio of protein to carbohydrate every time you eat. This one simple rule is the foundation for constructing a Zone-favorable diet. And what is that beneficial ratio of protein to carbohydrate? The ideal is about 0.75—that's three grams of protein to every four grams of carbohydrate.

That's the ideal. But there's a range of beneficial protein-to-carbohydrate ratios that are still Zone-favorable—between about 0.6 and 1.0 (see Figure 7-1). Not higher, not lower. (These numbers, by the way, are not based on animal research. They're based on the only species that counts: humans.)

The width of the range of the protein-to-carbohydrate ratio that allows you to enter the Zone depends on your genes. In this case, the genes that count are those that determine your insulin response to the carbohydrates you eat. Only 25 percent of the population has a favorably low insulin response. Everyone else's body responds to carbohydrates by producing too much insulin.

If you have a genetically low insulin response to carbohydrates, you're lucky. You can eat more carbohydrates and still maintain the protein-to-carbohydrate ratio you need to enter the Zone. In other words, you'll have a much wider variance or "slop factor" in the protein-to-carbohydrate ratio required to stay in the Zone than people

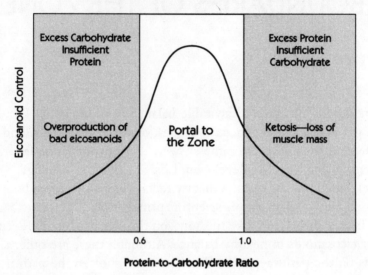

**Reaching the Zone Requires Precise Control
of the Protein-to-Carbohydrate Ratio**

Eicosanoid Control

Excess Carbohydrate
Insufficient
Protein

Excess Protein
Insufficient
Carbohydrate

Overproduction of
bad eicosanoids

Portal to
the Zone

Ketosis—loss of
muscle mass

0.6   1.0

Protein-to-Carbohydrate Ratio

Figure 7-1

who have less fortunate genes. This in turn will give you more leeway
before your body starts making excessive levels of bad eicosanoids.

On the other hand, if your genetic insulin response to carbohydrates is very high, the width of the range of your Zone-favorable
protein-to-carbohydrate ratio will be much narrower, and you'll have
a very low tolerance to even slight increases in the carbohydrate content of a meal or snack. So you'll have to be much more careful about
your carbohydrate intake, because your genetic "slop factor" is quite
low. It's not fair, but those are the genetic cards you were dealt. (By
the way, no matter what your genetics, as you age the "slop factor"
shrinks. So you can understand why it's so easy to put on weight as
you get older.)

In any case, even though your "slop factor" will be different, the
ideal protein-to-carbohydrate ratio will always be 0.75 (3g protein for
every 4 grams of carbohydrate) regardless of your genetics. This
means that at each meal you should eat a little more carbohydrate
than protein. That way you'll avoid ketosis, and still ensure that your
liver always has a store of carbohydrates big enough to maintain optimal brain function.

Regardless of your genetically determined insulin response to carbohydrates, the closer you get to the center of that ideal protein-to-carbohydrate ratio (0.75), the better your ability to control your balance of eicosanoids.

In fact, when you achieve the right mathematical ratio of protein-to-carbohydrate, you'll be able to control eicosanoids with druglike precision. In essence, you're treating food as if it were a prescription drug: delivering a controlled amount of protein and carbohydrate at every meal, and thus controlling the balance of eicosanoids for the next four to six hours. The better you control this eicosanoid balance, the better your quality of life.

THE PROTEIN FACTOR

Of course, the ideal protein-to-carbohydrate ratio is not just about carbohydrates. It's also about protein. Calories don't count, but protein does.

No one would ever advocate consuming more protein than your body requires. But likewise no one should ever advocate eating less protein than your body requires. Either extreme—too much or too little—can create serious health problems.

In Chapter 2 I explained what happens when you eat too much protein: you can induce ketosis, which ultimately means fat gain. But what happens if you eat too little protein? The result is a condition known as protein malnutrition. The symptoms of protein malnutrition include a weakened immune system, loss of muscle mass, and hair loss. But the most insidious effect of eating too little protein relative to carbohydrate is the overproduction of bad eicosanoids.

Although most experts contend that overt protein malnutrition is unusual in this country, it's less rare than you'd think. In fact, there are two groups in the American population who tend to be protein malnourished.

The first group includes anyone who's on a diet. Since protein-rich foods contain fat, most weight reduction diets tend to avoid protein. Supposedly, this will help decrease excess body fat. In reality removing large amounts of protein from the diet only promotes protein malnutrition. Since at least one-third of Americans are on a diet at any given time, this means that about one-third of Americans are also suffering from protein malnutrition.

Surprisingly, the second group of individuals who tend to be protein malnourished are elite athletes—especially women. Their protein demands are often exceedingly high because of their greater amounts of lean body mass and higher levels of physical activity. These hard-working athletes tend to consume more than enough calories, but they rarely eat adequate levels of protein.

So eating either too much protein or too little protein is unhealthy. All right, then: how much protein should you eat?

Most nutritionists like to assume that the protein needs of all men and women are uniform. We're told, for example, that every male needs 56 grams of protein per day, or that females require 45 grams per day. Unfortunately, the genetic and environmental diversity of humans make such simple-minded protein calculations meaningless. Fifty-six grams of protein may be adequate for a male who weighs 154 pounds, has 23 percent body fat (the average for American males), and is sedentary (unfortunately also average for American males). But if you're a male who happens to be larger, or have less body fat, or are more active, then that 56 grams of protein is not nearly enough to prevent protein malnutrition.

In reality, individual protein requirements are genetically different for every person on the face of the earth. One size does not fit all. In the next chapter, I'll show you how to calculate your personal protein requirement with precision and accuracy. For the moment I'd like you to give some thought to several other protein problems: where your protein is coming from, how much of that protein is getting into your bloodstream, and how fast it's getting there.

Here there is a difference between political correctness and hormonal correctness. Not all sources of protein are the same, and they don't all enter the bloodstream at the same rate. That's my concern: not the amount of protein you eat, but the amount that actually reaches the bloodstream, and the speed at which it gets there.

The amount of amino acids that actually enters the bloodstream is primarily determined by the digestibility of the protein source. If the enzymes of the digestive system can't get at the protein, the undigested protein simply passes through the system without being absorbed and used by the body.

Here's where fiber enters the game. The higher the fiber content of the protein source, the less its digestibility, and the less the body can absorb its constituent amino acids. It's as if there's a portion of the protein that you never ate at all.

Vegetable protein tends to be encased in a high-fiber network. Animal sources of protein have no fiber, and thus have a higher degree of digestibility. So vegetable sources of protein will not give the same gram-for-gram absorption of amino acids as animal-protein sources.

But there's a simple way to enhance significantly the digestibility—and thus the absorption rate—of vegetable protein. Just use isolated protein powders, in which the fiber has been stripped away by chemical processing. For vegetarians, this is an exceptionally important factor, since vegetarians want to get their protein from sources other than animals. It's easy to devise a diet that avoids meat and whole dairy products, but still supplies enough protein to satisfy the body's requirements for amino acids, including the essential amino acids. It simply means fortifying meals with vegetarian protein-rich sources such as tofu and isolated soybean protein powders.

So, whether you're a vegetarian or a meat eater, as long as you're getting your personal daily prescription of protein—and keeping that protein in the proper ratio relative to the carbohydrates you're eating—you'll have virtually equal access to the Zone.

DIETARY FASHION VERSUS THE ZONE-FAVORABLE DIET

As you'll see in the coming chapters, there's a good deal more to a Zone-favorable diet than just maintaining an ideal ratio of protein to carbohydrate. But as I said earlier, maintaining that ratio is the cardinal rule. So let's use that ratio as a basis to compare some currently popular diets with a diet that's Zone-favorable.

We'll start with the fashionable "healthy" diet that's recommended to virtually everybody in America—the diet that's low in fat, low in protein, and high in carbohydrates. If you're a cardiovascular patient or a world-class athlete, or if you're overweight, you probably follow this diet.

Figure 7-2 illustrates this recommended "healthy" diet. Notice that the carbohydrates in the recommended diet consist of primarily what I call unfavorable carbohydrates: lots of bread, pastas, rice, and potatoes. (You'll remember that these carbohydrates are unfavorable because they have a high glycemic index, and therefore a tendency to rapidly increase insulin levels.) The rest of the diet, almost as an after-thought, consists of 15 percent protein and 15 percent fat.

You might say, "That seems reasonable. That's what I see in the leading women's magazines, and they wouldn't lead me astray, any more than the medical journals or runners' magazines would. All these 'experts' can't be wrong."

But if you put the recommended "healthy" diet onto a pie chart as shown in Figure 7-2, it looks a little unbalanced—it looks like there's a large excess of carbohydrate. Still, the experts and the magazines all tell us that everyone should be eating this way.

How does the recommended healthy diet compare to a Zone-favorable diet (shown in Figure 7-3)? They're obviously very different.

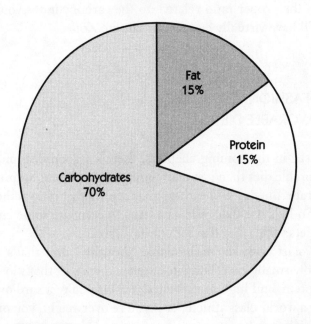

Caloric Composition of a Recommended "Healthy" Diet

Fat 15%

Protein 15%

Carbohydrates 70%

Figure 7-2

First of all, the Zone-favorable diet has a much lower carbohydrate percentage, and these carbohydrates are primarily the favorable low-glycemic variety: fruits and fiber-rich vegetables.

Still, if you're used to the recommended "healthy" diet, the Zone-favorable diet appears to have excessive levels of protein and lots of fat. You've been led to believe that if you follow such a diet, either you'll die of an immediate heart attack, or within a month you'll look like Porky Pig.

But now put the Zone-favorable diet on that same pie chart in Figure 7-3. Looks a little more balanced, doesn't it?

I make these two comparisons to point out that talking about diets in terms of the percentage of calories they supply from each macronutrient—and this is the way most diets are presented—is meaningless, at least as far as understanding the Zone is concerned.

Let me explain. Let's look at these diets, and a few others, in terms of the ratio of calories they supply from each of the macronutrients (see Figure 7-4). When you look at it this way—and if you

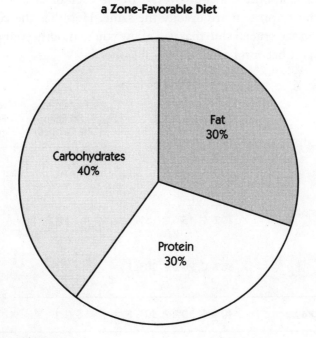

**Caloric Composition of
a Zone-Favorable Diet**

Fat
30%

Carbohydrates
40%

Protein
30%

Figure 7-3

look closely—you'll find that, surprisingly enough, they all have something in common. No matter how extreme each diet may appear to be, each one has the same percentage of calories coming from fat as from protein. Their protein-to-fat calorie ratio is always 1:1.

The vegetarian diet has 10 percent of its calories as protein and 10 percent of its calories as fat. The recommended "healthy" diet has 15 percent of its calories as protein and 15 percent of its calories as fat, again a one-to-one ratio. The American Diabetes Association diet has 20 percent of its calories as protein and 20 percent of calories as fat. Finally, the Zone-favorable diet has 30 percent of its calories as protein and 30 percent of its calories as fat, also maintaining the one-to-one ratio. So in each of these diets, which seem so radically different when compared to each other, there is a common denominator.

I've shown you this to illustrate my belief that in the world of nutrition nobody's really wrong. They just aren't quite correct. I always try to look for universalities in nutrition instead of controversies. If you look at the percent of calories in each of these diets, they appear to be totally divergent, with no connecting relationships. That divergence is a source of controversy. But in each of these diets, the ratios of fat to protein are exactly the same. Here lies the common linkage and the crucial clue that will allow you to modify your current diet so that it becomes a Zone-favorable diet.

Diet Comparisons

Diet	% Calories	Protein-to-Fat Ratio (% Calories)	Protein-to-Fat Ratio (Grams)
Vegetarian	80% C, 10% P, 10% F	1:1	1:0.4
Recommended "Healthy"	70% C, 15% P, 15% F	1:1	1:0.4
American Diabetes Assoc.	60% C, 20% P, 20% F	1:1	1:0.4
Zone-Favorable	40% C, 30% P, 30% F	1:1	1:0.4

Figure 7-4

But there's still another way to look at it. Fat contains nine calories per gram, while protein contains four calories per gram. This means that fat has 2.25 times more calories per gram than protein does. Therefore if we have a one-to-one ratio of calories for protein and fat in every diet, this also means that for every gram of protein you eat, you'd be eating slightly more than 0.4 of a gram of fat (it's actually 0.44)— regardless of the type of diet.

What pulls all this together? It's not the percentages of calories that each diet supplies. Once again: if you want to understand fully the hormonal effects of food, and therefore the Zone, it's meaningless to worry about the percentages of calories you're getting from each macronutrient. It's not the percent of calories that you put in your mouth; it's the absolute amounts, based on your protein require-ments, of macronutrients.

The real key to understanding a Zone-favorable diet is knowing your unique protein requirements. I'll use myself as an example, and see how my own personal protein requirement fits into each of the diets I've discussed.

I'm six feet five, moderately active, and not too overweight at 210. My daily protein requirement calculates to be 100 grams. If I eat any less than that amount of protein, I'll be protein malnourished. If I eat more than 100 grams of protein, that will be too much.

So take a look at Figure 7-5. I'm assuming that the amount of protein supplied by each of these diets is adequate. So whether I'm following the Zone-favorable diet, the American Diabetes Associa-tion diet, the recommended "healthy" diet, or the vegetarian diet, in each of these diets I should be consuming 100 grams of protein in the course of the day. And since we know that the amount of fat in grams is linked to the grams of protein in a strict ratio, then on each of these diets I'd be consuming exactly 44 grams of fat.

Surprise! In each of these diets, four seemingly very different diets, the absolute amount of protein and the amount of fat in grams that I should be consuming is exactly the same!

So what makes these diets different? Look at Figure 7-5 again. Using a Zone-favorable diet as a starting point for comparison, in the other diets I'm consuming increasing amounts of carbohydrates. More carbohydrates means more insulin. Too much insulin means too many bad eicosanoids. The end result: I'm pushed out of the

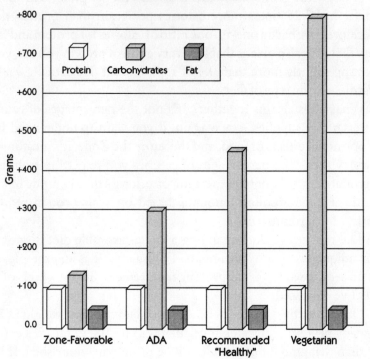

Figure 7-5

Zone. The further I am from the Zone, the fatter I become. The further I move away from the Zone, the more likely I am to become ill. The further I move away from the Zone, the poorer the quality of my life.

Another way to understand this concept is to graph each of these diets in terms of protein-to-carbohydrate ratios. The results are shown in Figure 7-6. As you can see, all the other diets have protein-to-carbohydrate ratios that are very low compared to a Zone-favorable diet. This means you can follow these diets forever, and you'll never reach the Zone.

Just for fun—and because it makes the comparison even more dramatic—I've thrown in some typical candy bars in Figure 7-6. Another surprise: these candy bars have almost the same protein-to-carbohydrate ratio as some of the diets! And guess what: in terms of macronutrient content, your digestive system can't tell the difference. In

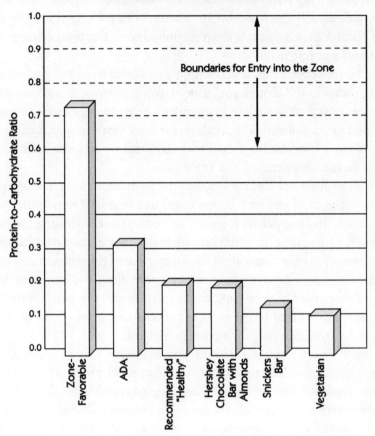

Figure 7-6

other words, many people following high-carbohydrate diets might just as well be eating candy bars.

I hope these comparisons will open your eyes to the value of using the protein-to-carbohydrate ratio (based on your unique protein requirements) as the centerpiece of your Zone-favorable diet. But what about total calories? After all, many diets are based on nothing more than cutting down your calorie consumption.

In the Zone, your total calorie needs don't change, but where they come from does. If you can meet a large portion of your calorie needs by more effectively accessing your internal stored body fat, then you don't have to put as many external calories in your mouth.

In fact, if you're in the Zone, your increased ability to use stored body fat to meet daily energy requirements will mean that your caloric intake will usually decrease by 50 percent. On a Zone-favorable diet you restrict excess calories from carbohydrates, not total calories and certainly not nutrition.

On the other hand, if you shut down access to stored body fat by being outside the Zone, you have to keep putting more and more calories into your mouth to maintain adequate energy levels required for basic metabolism. More calories means more food. Outside the Zone, more food means excess body fat. And we all know that excess body fat means increased risk of disease.

Let's sum it up. Remember that the foundation for a Zone-favorable diet is drug-delivery technology, not standard nutritional prescriptions. In drug delivery, the major concern is controlling the rates of entry of the drug into the bloodstream. In a Zone-favorable diet, the primary goal is controlling the entry rates of protein and carbohydrate into the bloodstream, thereby controlling the resulting hormonal responses. Controlling those rates of entry means always trying to maintain that target ratio of protein-to-carbohydrate between 0.6 and 1.0, with an ideal target ratio of 0.75.

In the next chapter I'll show you how easy it is to make Zone-favorable meals and snacks that have this ideal protein-to-carbohydrate ratio built in. If you eat these Zone-favorable meals on a consistent basis, your reward is a desirable balance of eicosanoids. That favorable balance of eicosanoids spells optimal health.

To put it in one sentence, a Zone-favorable diet is a protein-adequate, low-fat, moderate-carbohydrate program. Not a very radical diet after all. In fact, it's very similar to the diet recommended by your grandmother—even if she knew nothing about eicosanoids and the Zone.

CHAPTER EIGHT

YOUR DIETARY ROAD MAP TO THE ZONE

I've said this before, but it's worth saying again: If you want to permanently reap the rewards of living in the Zone, you have to make a radical change in the way you think about food. Food is far more important than just something you eat for pleasure or to appease your hunger. Rather, it is a potent drug that you'll take at least three times a day for the rest of your life. Once food is broken down into its basic components (glucose, amino acids, and fatty acids) and sent into the bloodstream, *it has a more powerful impact on your body—and your health—than any drug your doctor could ever prescribe.*

Every time you eat, you are taking very strong medicine, which can have a good, bad, or indifferent effect on your body for the next four to six hours. When a doctor prescribes a pill, he doesn't tell you to take all the pills the first day—that would overload your system, and might even kill you. Instead, the doctor wants you to maintain moderate but relatively constant levels of that drug in your bloodstream over the course of the treatment.

Every drug has a therapeutic zone. Too much of the drug in the bloodstream can bring on a toxic reaction, too little can make the drug ineffective. For the drug to work, you have to maintain the right level in the bloodstream. So it's not just the drug that treats your condition and restores your health, it's also the consistency and moderation of the dose—in other words, staying within that therapeutic zone.

The same is true of food. The key is to maintain a consistently healthful balance of eicosanoids over the longest possible period of time. Every meal and every snack you eat should have the desired balance of macronutrients—protein, carbohydrates, and fats—that produces an appropriate and favorable hormone response, especially in terms of glucagon, insulin, and the eicosanoids.

So don't focus on calories—especially percentages of calories. As I've already pointed out, that's a meaningless concept. Once again, here's the primary prescription that will allow you to get to the center of the Zone: make sure you know how much protein you require, and maintain the ratio of protein to carbohydrate as close to 0.75 as possible—every meal, every snack, every day.

This guideline is easy to follow. In many ways maintaining this protein-to-carbohydrate ratio is no different from maintaining the ideal combustion mixture of gas and air for your car's engine. It takes only a relatively minor adjustment in your current dietary habits. But that minor adjustment in the macronutrient composition of your meals will produce major rewards in terms of your overall health and well-being.

Since the stakes are so very high, it's important to make that adjustment carefully, with an eye toward accuracy. But it's not hard. To reach the Zone, all you have to do is follow the easy rules I'm about to describe.

THE PROTEIN PRESCRIPTION

The first step in building a Zone-favorable diet is to know your daily protein requirement. The amount of protein that you require will be genetically unique to you and you alone. (When I say protein, I don't necessarily mean eating more meat. From a drug-delivery viewpoint, I don't care if your protein comes from a canister of protein powder, a slice of turkey, or a piece of tofu.) No matter what the protein source, the correct amount of protein depends upon only three factors: your weight, your percentage of body fat, and your level of physical activity.

To determine your unique protein requirement, start by computing your percentage of body fat. Everyone knows their weight, but virtually no one knows their percentage of body fat. Well, you can determine that number quite easily, using the worksheets in Appendix B. The only tools you'll need are a scale, a tape measure, and a pencil.

By simply taking specific measurements at specific locations on your body (these locations, you'll notice, are different for men and women), you can calculate your percentage of body fat and your lean body mass. The beauty of this approach is that measurements can be done frequently and easily in the privacy of your own home. More important, if you're trying to lose weight, you can recalculate your percentage of body fat as time goes on to see the progress you've made.

Once you know your percentage of body fat, using the formulas in Appendix E, you can easily calculate your total fat-mass and your lean body mass. (You might also wish to see a comparison of body-fat percentage among different groups of people. If so, refer to Appendix F.)

The other half of the protein-requirement equation is your level of physical activity. How active are you? Do you spend all day watching Donahue and Oprah? Or do you spend four hours a day in the pool like the Stanford University swimmers? The higher your physical-activity level, the faster the rate that you're breaking down protein. As a result, you'll need to increase your dietary protein intake to repair and rebuild muscle that gets damaged during higher levels of physical activity.

These activity factors are listed below.

If you're sedentary, you'll need only 0.5 grams of protein per pound of lean body mass to maintain that lean body mass. If you're doing heavy weight workouts every day or exercising twice a day, you'll need twice that amount (1.0 grams of protein per pound of lean body mass). Between those two extremes lies a continuum. If you're significantly overweight (greater than 30 percent of body fat for males and 40 percent of body fat for females), you're inadvertently doing light weight training twenty-four hours per day, so give yourself a 0.6 activity factor. (This quasi-weight training for obese individuals is the reason they usually have more lean body mass than thin people. Overweight people simply require more muscle to carry the added weight. Unfortunately, they also have far greater amounts of stored fat.)

Now you're ready to calculate your protein requirements. Remember: they're unique to you and no one else.

To show you how easy it is to make these calculations, let's take the mythical 154-pound male—the guy who's so often paraded by nutritionists as the standard for adequate protein intake. Let's also

TABLE 8-1

Physical-Activity Factors

ACTIVITY	PROTEIN REQUIREMENTS (GRAMS PER POUND OF LEAN BODY MASS)
Sedentary	0.5
Light (i.e., walking)	0.6
Moderate (30 minutes per day, 3 times per week)	0.7
Active (1 hour per day, 5 times per week)	0.8
Very active (2 hours per day, 5 times per week)	0.9
Heavy weight training or twice-a-day exercise (5 days per week)	1.0

TABLE 8-2

Calculating Your Protein Requirements

_____ Your Lean Body Mass (LBM) (from Appendix B)

× _____ Your Activity Factor (from Table 8-1)

= _____ Your Daily Protein Requirement

assume that this mythical 154-pound male has 23 percent body fat (the average for American males) and is sedentary (also, unfortunately, an excellent assumption for the average American male).

Using the above formulas, this mythical 154-pound male would have 36 pounds of total fat (154 pounds times 0.23 equals 36 pounds of fat). With this amount of total fat, he would have 118 pounds of lean body mass (154 pounds of total weight minus 36 pounds of total fat). Multiplying this lean body mass by 0.5 grams protein per pound of lean body mass (the activity factor for a sedentary individual) gives this mythical 154-pound male a daily protein requirement of 59 grams (118 pounds times 0.5 grams per pound equals 59).

This figure is virtually identical to the 56 grams of daily protein recommended for everyone by the National Academy of Sciences. Isn't science wonderful? But not everyone is the mythical 154-pound male. I'm definitely not. My protein requirements using the above formulas is 100 grams of protein per day. That's the amount I should eat—no more, no less.

Once you know your protein requirement, you can begin to treat that total protein requirement as a prescription drug. That means spreading your intake of protein evenly throughout the day, just as you would with any prescribed medication.

Let's say your protein requirement is 75 grams a day. Don't try to get it all by eating steak and eggs for breakfast. Besides stuffing yourself with two protein sources rich in arachidonic acid (the building block of bad eicosanoids), you will also be overloading the body's capacity for protein utilization at that particular meal.

Remember that even though protein primarily stimulates glucagon, it also has an effect on insulin. Taking in too much protein at a meal will increase insulin levels, and begin to take you out of the Zone. Furthermore, if you consume too much protein in one meal, you have a tendency to reduce the amount of protein in other meals. As a result, other meals will have relatively little protein to counteract the carbohydrates you'll be eating. Again your insulin-glucagon balance will tip toward the insulin side, and your eicosanoid balance will be thrown off in the opposite direction. You'll drive yourself out of the Zone.

Spread your protein requirement evenly throughout the day, over three meals and two snacks. To make it easy, follow my *macronutrient block method*. Think of your total protein requirements as protein blocks, each block consisting of 7 grams of protein. If your daily protein requirement is, say, 75 grams, then this would be equivalent to 11 protein blocks (simply round off to the nearest whole number). Try eating three protein blocks at each of your three meals, and one protein block at each of your two snacks—late afternoon and before bedtime.

So here's what a typical day might look like when divided into protein blocks:

Breakfast	Lunch	Late afternoon snack	Dinner	Late night snack
3 P	3 P	1 P	3 P	1 P

Spreading your protein requirement throughout the day means following another important rule: Never go more than five hours without eating a Zone-favorable meal or Zone-favorable snack. Remember that the hormonal effects of a meal will last only four to six hours. But you want to keep yourself in the Zone, not just for four to six hours, but throughout the day. This means that even after you've reached the Zone you have to repeat this process every four to six hours with a meal or snack. In essence, you're only as good hormonally as your last meal, and you are only as good hormonally as your next meal.

The minimum amount of protein required to restart the process is one block. So let's start with three protein blocks at breakfast. If you eat breakfast at seven o'clock, then plan to eat lunch no later than twelve o'clock (remember the five-hour rule). At lunch, eat three protein blocks. Since most people eat dinner at seven o'clock at night, that will be too long between meals, so eat a late-afternoon snack at about five o'clock. That snack should contain one protein block.

At dinner, eat another three-protein block. Before you go to bed, eat a late-night snack containing one protein block. (Why a late-night snack? You're going on an eight-hour fast and you want to stay in the Zone while you sleep.) The next morning, you simply start again.

Following this program, you've consumed your eleven blocks of protein, and you've spread them throughout the day, just as you would a drug. Of course, if your protein requirements were higher or lower than 75 grams, then the number of protein blocks you'd eat during the day would also be higher or lower.

Table 8-3 lists the quantities of typical low-fat protein sources containing one block of protein. Whatever number a meal requires in protein blocks, simply add enough protein blocks together to get to that number. Remember: if your breakfast requirement is three protein blocks but you've only eaten two, you have to make it up by adding a protein block to one of your other meals or snacks during the day.

TABLE 8-3

Typical Protein Blocks

Listed below are some typical amounts of protein-rich but low-fat choices, each containing one block of protein (approximately seven grams). A more complete listing can be found in Appendix C.

Animal Sources

Skinless chicken breast (1 oz.)   Turkey breast (1 oz.)

Lean pork (1 oz.)   Lean lamb (1 oz.)

Fish Sources

Cod (1.5 oz.)   Tuna (1 oz.)

Shrimp (1.5 oz.)   Salmon (1.5 oz.)

Egg Sources

Egg whites (2)   Egg Beaters (¼ cup)

Vegetarian Sources

Tofu (3 oz.)   Protein powder (1/3 oz.)

Dairy Sources

Low-fat cottage cheese (2 oz.)

CARBOHYDRATES

Once you know your daily protein requirement in blocks, it becomes easy to determine how much carbohydrate you should eat. For every protein block at a meal or snack, simply make sure that you eat one carbohydrate block.

Remember that one protein block contains 7 grams. Since one carbohydrate block is 9 grams, at each meal or snack you're consuming a little more carbohydrate than protein—but not much more. Maintaining the protein and carbohydrate blocks in a one-to-one ratio will always generate the desired protein-to-carbohydrate ratio of about 0.75, and that ratio positions you squarely in the middle of the Zone.

As an example, let's use the protein requirement of 75 grams a day, rounded off to 11 protein blocks. If that's your total protein requirement, then you should also be eating 11 carbohydrate blocks over the course of a day. And just as you did with protein, you should spread your carbohydrate requirement evenly through each of the day's meals and snacks. Just think of balance.

Now your daily meal plan would look like this:

Breakfast	Lunch	Late afternoon snack	Dinner	Late night snack
3 P	3 P	1 P	3 P	1 P
3 C	3 C	1 C	3 C	1 C

Now comes another important Zone rule. *Be especially careful about the types of carbohydrates you eat.* All carbohydrates are not equal. Favorable carbohydrates usually have a low glycemic index—they enter the bloodstream slowly, raise blood-sugar levels slowly, and produce a moderate insulin response. This means they maintain a favorable balance of eicosanoids, and that keeps you in the Zone.

Unfavorable carbohydrates generally have a high glycemic index—they enter the bloodstream quickly, raise blood-sugar levels quickly, and produce an exaggerated insulin response. (This is the biochemical cause of carbohydrate cravings.) An elevated insulin response will tilt your eicosanoid balance toward the negative, and you'll be pushed out of the Zone. So unfavorable carbohydrates should be used in moderation, and in much smaller amounts than favorable carbohydrates.

(Another reason to keep your consumption of unfavorable carbohydrates moderate is that these foods are extremely carbohydrate-dense. As such, they rapidly use up your total carbohydrate-block allotment for a meal and for the day. By the way, if you do eat unfavorable carbohydrates—especially bread—always use whole-grain versions.)

So you want to make sure that most of your carbohydrate blocks consist of favorable carbohydrates. These include most—although not all—fiber-rich fruits and vegetables. Unfavorable carbohydrates include bread, pasta, grains, corn, potatoes, and high-glycemic fruits and vegetables, like papayas, bananas, corn, and carrots—as well as fruit juices.

Table 8-4 lists many of the favorable and unfavorable carbohydrates, and gives you typical serving sizes per carbohydrate block. A more complete listing can be found in Appendix C. (Again, remember that one carbohydrate block contains about nine grams of carbohydrate.)

FATS

To complete a Zone-favorable meal, always add fat. Remember, you're trying to use every trick in the book from a drug-delivery perspective to achieve a favorable balance of eicosanoids on a consistent basis. Using fat is one of those tricks.

Here's how the trick works: Besides supplying the building blocks for eicosanoids, fats also function as another control rod, just like fiber, to slow the entry rate of carbohydrates into the bloodstream.

Fats are also important for two other reasons. First, they make food taste better. A truly boring diet is a fat-free diet—ask any French chef. The second reason is that the fat content in a meal causes the release of a hormone called *cholecystokinin* (CCK) from the stomach. That hormone tells the brain that you're satisfied, and to stop eating.

So don't be afraid of fats: they're vital to eicosanoid production, and essential for reducing excess body fat, as well as generating overall good health.

But, you say, if most protein sources also contain fat, why should I add fat blocks to my meals? Even though low-fat protein sources do contain some fat, it's not the ideal amount of fat you need to get to the center of the Zone. To get that ideal amount, you'll need to add some extra fat blocks. (Don't get the wrong idea: this is not an invitation to fat gluttony. You're not going to spend your day gobbling up lard.)

When you add those fat blocks, though, you must pay careful attention to the *kind* of fat you eat. Just as there are favorable and unfavorable carbohydrates, there are also good fats and bad fats.

What are bad fats? The real villain fat is arachidonic acid, the chemical building block for all bad eicosanoids. This is the one fat you should definitely try to restrict, if not eliminate, from your diet. (In later chapters I'll tell you why in more detail.) Food sources high in arachidonic acid are egg yolks, organ meats (like liver and most deli

TABLE 8-4

Typical Carbohydrate Blocks

Favorable Carbohydrates

COOKED VEGETABLES (FRESH OR FROZEN)	RAW VEGETABLES
1 cup (12 spears) cooked asparagus	2 cups broccoli or cauliflower
1 cup broccoli	2 cups shredded cabbage
¼ cup lentils, kidney beans, etc.	1 large tomato
1½ cups cauliflower	1 head lettuce
1 cup green or wax beans	4 cups spinach
1 cup zucchini	3 cups sliced cucumber
	2 cups celery
	2 green peppers

FRUITS	
½ medium apple	1 peach
½ medium orange	½ medium grapefruit
½ cup cherries (7 cherries)	½ cup grapes (9 grapes)
3 apricots	1 kiwi
½ large nectarine	¼ cantaloupe
⅓ medium pear	1 medium plum
1 cup strawberries	1 tangerine
½ cup pineapple, cubed	½ cup blueberries

Unfavorable Carbohydrates

⅕ cup brown rice	½ slice bread
¼ cup pasta	¼ bagel
½ cup papaya	½ 6-inch flour tortilla
⅓ cup mango	2 carrots
⅓ banana	
½ oz. dry breakfast cereal	

FRUIT JUICES

Apple juice (3 oz.)
Grapefruit juice (4 oz.)
Orange juice (4 oz.)

meats), and fatty red meat. Obviously you want to keep these foods to a minimum or restrict them entirely.

Saturated fats should also be kept to a minimum. Saturated fats are found in animal protein sources and in whole-fat dairy products. You want to restrict these fats in a Zone-favorable diet because they tend to raise insulin levels by creating a condition known as *insulin resistance*. (I'll explain this condition in detail in the chapter on heart disease.) Although not nearly as bad as arachidonic acid, saturated fats are still not desirable. Try to limit your consumption of them. That's why I recommend low-fat animal protein sources like white meat poultry and fish—they're low in saturated fat.

Are there "good" fats? Of course. Most of the good fats are monounsaturated fats—those found in olive oil, canola oil, olives, macadamia nuts, and avocados (and of course guacamole). (A diet rich in monounsaturated fats is sometimes called a Mediterranean diet.)

Monounsaturated fatty acids are eicosanoid neutral. They can't be converted into eicosanoids (good or bad), and they have no effect on insulin levels. Since you've spent so much time adjusting your pro-tein-to-carbohydrate ratio to control insulin, monounsaturated fats should be the major source of fat in your diet—that way, you'll avoid disrupting the delicate hormonal balance you've worked to achieve.

To sum up, then, here's the Zone rule on fat: restrict bad fats—arachidonic acid and saturated fat—and get most of your daily fat in-take from good (monounsaturated) fat.

Table 8-5 gives some examples of good fats (a more complete list can be found in Appendix C). Each example makes up one fat block, and each fat block contains approximately 1 1/2 grams of fat. Actu-ally, that's not much fat at all—remember, a Zone-favorable diet *is* a low-fat diet.

Now that you know what kind of fat to eat, the question is how much. That's easy: for every protein block in a meal or snack, just add one fat block. That gives you the ideal ratio at each meal and each

TABLE 8-5

Typical Fat Blocks

3 olives*   ⅓ teaspoon olive oil*

⅓ teaspoon canola oil*   1 macadamia nut*

                                    ½ teaspoon natural peanut butter*

1 teaspoon light mayonnaise

½ teaspoon mayonnaise

---

*rich in monounsaturated fat

snack, based solely on your protein needs. And just as you did with protein and carbohydrate, spread the fat intake evenly throughout the day, so the ratio of protein, carbohydrate and fat blocks is always maintained at 1:1:1 at every meal or snack. (Note: Truly elite athletes should consume two fat blocks for every protein block. Therefore their ratio of protein, carbohydrate, and fat blocks would be 1:1:2. The extra fat is needed because of their intensive training, but this fat should be almost all monounsaturated fat.)

For a person whose protein requirement is eleven blocks per day, a Zone-favorable program would now look like this:

Breakfast	Lunch	Late afternoon snack	Dinner	Late night snack
3 P	3 P	1 P	3 P	1 P
3 C	3 C	1 C	3 C	1 C
3 F	3 F	1 F	3 F	1 F

This program combines the proper amounts of protein and carbohydrates with the proper amount of fat to maintain insulin and glucagon secretion at optimal levels. In shorthand, that means a favorable balance of eicosanoids: a day spent in the Zone.

Now let's put it all together, so you can see how easy it is to build a Zone-favorable meal. To start, simply round off your protein requirement for each meal to the nearest whole number of protein blocks. Then add an equivalent number of carbohydrate and fat blocks, and you're done.

What about Zone-favorable snacks? Use the same calculations. Listed in Table 8-6 are some representative samples. Each of these snacks contains approximately one block each of protein, carbohydrate, and fat. (For more Zone-favorable snacks, see Appendix D.)

TABLE 8-6

Zone-favorable Snacks

¼ cup low-fat cottage cheese plus ½ piece of fruit
4 oz. plain low-fat yogurt *without* any added fruit or other carbohydrate
6 oz. low-fat milk

So let's review our Zone-favorable diet construction project, again using the person who requires 75 grams of protein a day as an example. Remember, this person is eating three meals containing three protein blocks and two snacks with one protein block each. So this person would simply choose three protein blocks, then add three carbohydrate blocks, and three fat blocks. Sort of like ordering at a Chinese restaurant, except in this case, presto: you have a Zone-favorable meal.

What about the snacks? Simply choose one from Table 8-6 to make up your own.

What if you want to add more protein blocks to a meal? Simply add the same number of carbohydrate and fat blocks to keep everything in balance. It's easy if you pay attention.

There's one caveat, though. Even if you have a perfectly balanced Zone meal, if you eat more protein blocks in a day than your body requires, you'll end up consuming more protein than you need. Remember that any excess protein that the body can't immediately use will be turned into fat. This will slow down your rate of fat loss, and even potentially drive you out of the Zone.

Also, excess protein blocks mean excess calories. If you consume too many calories at a meal, insulin levels will rise, and that means overproduction of bad eicosanoids. What you're trying to achieve is a precise ratio of protein to carbohydrate, *keeping the total calories at any one meal to 500 or less—100 or less for snacks.* This means you should never eat more than six protein blocks per meal, as these would exceed this calorie limit. (A typical meal with four protein blocks and of course the same number of carbohydrate blocks and fat blocks would total less than 400 calories.)

That combination—low-calorie meals with the right combination of protein, carbohydrate, and fat blocks—will keep you in the Zone for the next four to six hours. So, if you can add simple numbers, you can construct Zone-favorable meals for the rest of your life, using only the foods you like, and by making only subtle changes in your eating style. In other words, you don't have to make a radical change in your diet. Just apply the Zone rules to the way you currently eat. I think you'll agree that this is an extraordinarily flexible program.

Here's another way to look at it: think of your Zone-favorable meal or snack as a construction project. Pretend you're building a house. The protein blocks are your foundation, and they determine how high the superstructure of carbohydrate blocks can be before it topples over into a pool of excess insulin. Carbohydrate blocks are the walls of the house, and fat blocks are the roof. If you've built your house (i.e., meal) properly, you're going to be in the Zone. It's that simple.

For example, if a meal contains:

—2 blocks of protein, add 2 blocks of carbohydrate and 2 blocks of fat
—3 blocks of protein, add 3 blocks of carbohydrate and 3 blocks of fat
—4 blocks of protein, add 4 blocks of carbohydrate and 4 blocks of fat
—5 blocks of protein, add 5 blocks of carbohydrate and 5 blocks of fat
—6 blocks of protein, add 6 blocks of carbohydrate and 6 blocks of fat

As I said, my macronutrient block method is an easy way to make Zone-favorable meals. If you can add, you can follow this program. But if you don't want to make these calculations yourself, just turn to the Appendix in the back of the book. Here you'll find a series of meals and recipes in which the proper macronutrient proportions have already been set. In other words, the math's been done for you. Or you can use the Easy Eyeball Method outlined later in this chapter.

As a sample, though, I'd like to show you what all these numbers mean when you translate them into real meals in the real world. I'd like to show you that these Zone-favorable meals actually taste good. So here are some Zone-favorable recipes, courtesy of French-trained professional chef Jeanette Pothier and her colleague Anne Rislove.

Each recipe contains four protein blocks, four carbohydrate blocks, and four fat blocks. Additional recipes—enough for a week's worth of Zone-favorable meals—can be found in Appendix D.

TURKEY ESCALOPES FONTINA
(serves 4)

12 ounces thin-sliced turkey breast
½ teaspoon olive oil
1 teaspoon butter
Salt and pepper
2 cloves garlic
15 sprigs parsley
½ cup chicken stock
1 ounce Fontina cheese, shredded

Pound the turkey slices with a meat pounder until they are as thin as possible.

Heat the olive oil in a large skillet and add the butter. When it has melted, sauté the turkey a few slices at a time until they are lightly browned. Remove them to a buttered ovenproof dish, sprinkle with salt and pepper, and keep them hot.

Turn on the broiler. Fit a food processor with the steel blade and halve the garlic cloves. With the machine running, drop in the garlic and then quickly add the parsley. Alternatively you can chop them very fine by hand.

Add the garlic and parsley to the oil in the skillet, and add half the chicken stock. Bring it to a boil, scraping the bottom of the pan well to remove any sediment. Then add the remaining stock and reduce the mixture by half. Pour this sauce over the turkey slices.

Sprinkle the turkey with the cheese, and broil just to melt the cheese. Serve at once with Vegetable "Pasta" (see Appendix D).

4 protein blocks per serving

BREAKFAST BURRITOS
(serves 6)

8 ounces Jimmy Dean turkey sausage
8 ounces shredded potatoes
1½ cups egg substitute
¼ cup picante sauce
6 corn tortillas
6 ounces Mexican cheese

Remove the sausage from the package and break it up with a fork. Spray a 9-inch skillet with olive oil. Over medium heat, cook the sausage until it just begins to turn gray. Peel the potatoes and shred them. Dry them in a tea towel to remove some of the moisture. Add these potatoes to the skillet and toss well to mix. Cook, tossing frequently until the potatoes turn translucent, approximately 8 to 10 minutes. Add the egg substitute and stir into the mixture. Using a flat wooden spatula, turn the mixture until the eggs are cooked. Add the picante sauce and mix well. Remove from the heat.

Meanwhile, cut 6 pieces of foil, each large enough to hold a tortilla. Place one tortilla on each piece, and divide the sausage-and-egg mixture into 6 portions. Spread a portion over each tortilla and roll it, ending with the fold underneath. Wrap in the foil until ready to use, or freeze.

To eat, remove the foil, and place the burritos on a microwave-safe plate. Add picante sauce and 1 ounce of cheese for each. Microwave just until the cheese melts.

Finish with 4 ounces orange juice diluted with another 4 ounces of spring water.

4 protein blocks per serving

NEW ENGLAND BOUILLABAISSE
(serves 4)

10 ounces leeks, cut in half, sliced thin, and washed under running
    water
15 ounces chicken broth
8 1-inch-diameter red potatoes, peeled and cut in half
4 ounces lobster meat
4 ounces bay scallops, cleaned and side muscle removed
4 ounces raw shrimp, cleaned and shelled
6 ounces clams (8-10 shelled or canned whole clams)
8 ounces canned tomatoes
3 ⅓ cups water
1 fish garnish
3 tablespoons unsalted butter

Place the leeks and half the chicken broth in a heavy soup pot. Cook
for 10 to 15 minutes over medium heat, stirring often. Add the rest of
the broth and the potatoes and bring back to a boil, then test the
potatoes for doneness. Add the clams and shrimp and just before it
boils again, add the scallops. Cook until they turn opaque. Add the
lobster and butter and turn off the heat. Add salt or pepper in moderation.

Serve with one small cornbread muffin apiece.

4 protein blocks per serving

I think you'll find that the recipes, both here and in the Appendix,
are extremely satisfying and full of flavor. And, of course, they'll get
you to the Zone.

SHOPPING IN THE ZONE

It's easy to shop in the Zone: just stay on the perimeter of the supermarket, and rarely go down the aisles. The food aisles are nothing
more than one large carbohydrate divided up into different packages,
all of them beckoning you to take them home and gobble them up.

To calculate the macronutrient content of the prepared food

products you're using—especially if you're buying frozen meals—review the Nutrition Facts on the label. These are your greatest ally. Calculate how many protein blocks and carbohydrate blocks there are in a serving size (remember that a protein block is seven grams, a carbohydrate block is nine grams). If the blocks aren't in a 1:1 ratio, that packaged food will never get you to the Zone. To bring a prepared food to the correct ratio, you may have to add some extra low-fat protein. (A listing of Zone-favorable dinners can be found in Appendix D.)

When buying fresh foods, you can always use the following guideline as a general rule of thumb:

—4 ounces of low-fat meat contain approximately 4 blocks of protein
—6 ounces of fish contain approximately 4 blocks of protein
—2 cups of raw vegetables contain approximately 1 block of carbohydrate
—1 piece of fruit contains approximately 2 blocks of carbohydrate
—1 cup of cooked pasta, beans, or rice contains approximately 4 blocks of carbohydrate

THE EYEBALL METHOD

If the thought of weighing and measuring all the food you eat, or even reading food labels, makes you groan—or if you're simply too busy to pay careful attention to weights and measures—don't worry. You can formulate a Zone-favorable meal just by using your eyeballs. Although not as precise as my macronutrient block method, with time and practice your eyesight can become a pretty good calculator.

Start with the protein, using the palm of your hand as a guide. The amount of protein that can fit into your palm is usually four protein blocks. That's about one chicken breast or 4 ounces sliced turkey.

The size of the protein on your plate will help you determine the size of your carbohydrate portions. If you're eating favorable carbohydrates, then the size of your carbohydrate portion should be about twice as big as your protein portion. If you're eating unfavorable carbohydrates, make that carbohydrate portion the same size as your protein portion.

If you plan to have some dessert—most desserts are almost all carbohydrate—simply cut back on the amount of carbohydrates you eat on the plate.

If your protein source is low-fat—and it should be—then you can get the rest of the fat you need by adding some salad dressing to a side salad, or a small amount of mayonnaise, or eating a few olives.

RESTAURANT EATING IN THE ZONE

In this high-speed day and age, few people eat all their meals at home. And for anyone trying to follow a nutritional prescription, restaurant eating can be a real challenge, if not a downright obstacle. What do you do when you eat out?

First, before you go out try to eat a Zone-favorable snack. Once you reach the restaurant, don't eat the rolls (easier if you had that snack before going out). More important, you want to save some of your carbohydrate blocks for dessert at the end of the meal.

Order a low-fat entrée. When it arrives, eyeball how much protein you have on your plate—again, using the palm of your hand as a measuring guide. Use the eyeball method again to determine the size of your carbohydrate portion on your plate. Remember, it doesn't matter how much of each macronutrient the restaurant serves you— what matters is how much you actually eat. So if you're planning to have dessert, make a mental note to cut back on the carbohydrates you eat with your entrée. If you plan to have a glass of wine, cut back your carbohydrate intake even further.

At the end of the meal, when the waiter comes back and asks the question "Any dessert?" your response is an immediate yes, to the shock of your dinner companions. Well, you saved up your carbohydrate blocks at dinner, now it's time to cash in. Order a dessert, and then ask, "Does anyone want half?" You eat your half of the dessert, and remain in the Zone.

So you've gone out to your favorite restaurant, and you've had a great dinner—a nice piece of protein, a little carbohydrate, a glass of fine wine, and half an extraordinary dessert. When it's all over, you're still in the Zone. Life is good!

THE DRIVE-THRU ZONE

Of course, the biggest challenge of all is the fast-food restaurant. Believe it or not, you can still construct Zone-favorable meals—and remain in "the Zone"—even when under the golden arches. In fact, if you order wisely, fast-food items can provide a nearly ideal ratio of protein to carbohydrate for an occasional quick meal on the run.

If you don't believe me, just turn to Appendix D. You'll find a complete list of Zone-favorable menu entrées from a wide variety of fast-food restaurants.

RULES OF THE ROAD TO REACH THE ZONE

Now let's put it all together. The rules of the road are simple:

1. Know how much protein your body needs. Never consume more protein than your body requires. And never consume less.
2. Every time you eat, make sure you maintain a 1:1 ratio of protein to carbohydrate blocks.
3. Spread your protein requirement throughout the day in three small Zone-favorable meals and two Zone-favorable snacks.
4. Never let more than five hours pass without eating a Zone-favorable meal or snack. (You're only as good as your last meal, and you're only as good as your next meal. The best time to eat is when you aren't hungry.)
5. Make your protein choices low-fat.
6. Make your carbohydrate choices from favorable carbohydrates (fiber-rich vegetables and fruits).
7. Make your fat choices from monounsaturated fats.
8. Try not to eat more than 500 calories per meal or 100 calories per snack. If your protein requirements are exceptionally high (for instance, if you're an NFL football player), you'll have to eat more than three meals per day.

HELPFUL HINTS FOR THE ZONE

As with any technology, there are some hints that will help you reach the Zone:

1. If you don't build a meal with the precise ratio of protein to carbohydrate blocks, don't panic. A slightly higher or lower protein-to-carbohydrate ratio will still get you closer to the Zone. You just won't find yourself directly in the center, where eicosanoid balance is ideal. If you want to reach the center of the Zone, the responsibility is yours.

2. Remember that this is not a calorie-deprivation program. In fact, you may have trouble eating all the food required to reach the Zone.

3. Your goal is to spend as much time in the Zone as possible. So plan your daily dietary strategy based on your wake-up time, then determine the points throughout the day when you'll need to fuel your body. In other words, treat food as if it were a prescribed medication.

4. Always drink at least 8 ounces of water or a sugar-free decaffeinated beverage with every meal or snack. If you are a heavy caffeine user, gradually reduce caffeine intake to zero whenever possible. (The breakdown products of caffeine will tend to increase insulin levels, and thus drive you out of the Zone.)

5. If you find yourself hungry and craving sugar or sweets two to three hours after a meal, you probably consumed too many carbohydrates that last meal. Whenever you have a problem with hunger or carbohydrate cravings, look to your last meal for a clue to the reason why.

6. No matter how consistently you follow this dietary strategy, you are bound to make mistakes. This is especially true at parties or when traveling. Remember, if you're only out of the Zone for a short period of time, you're only one meal away from reentering. It's like falling off a bike—you just get back up and continue your journey.

Now that you know the rules for reaching the Zone, you finally have a dietary road map for the rest of your life. Remember: a single Zone-favorable meal will give you four to six hours in the Zone. A day of Zone-favorable meals is a day in the Zone, and a lifetime of Zone-favorable meals is a lifetime in the Zone. The choice is yours.

So *bon appétit*, and welcome to the Zone!

CHAPTER NINE

EVOLUTION AND THE ZONE

If you follow a Zone-favorable diet consistently, you'll soon experience sweeping changes in the way you feel—physically, mentally, even emotionally. Why are these changes so broad, and at the same time so basic? Because from an evolutionary point of view—that is, a genetic point of view—*this is the way human beings are designed to eat.*

To understand that statement, we need to take a trip backward in evolutionary time. Start about 500 million years ago. At that point, of course, *Homo sapiens* as a species was nowhere to be seen—-in fact, it would be another 495 million years (give or take a million or so) before the first protohumans would evolve.

Humans weren't around, but eicosanoids were. In fact, *eicosanoids represented one of the first hormonal control systems for living organisms to interact with their environment.* This is why some of the eicosanoids that sponges make are the same ones that humans make today. This is why every living cell in the human body is capable of making eicosanoids, as the ability of an individual cell to make an eicosanoid has been conserved during the last 500 million years of evolution.

So first came the eicosanoids. About 450 million years later came the appearance of paired endocrine hormones like insulin and glucagon, hormones that require a secreting gland and use of the bloodstream to reach their target tissues. These hormones required a preexisting biological control system to regulate them, and since eicosanoids were already around, eicosanoids got the job. In that sense, eicosanoids represented the central processing unit that controls virtually all other hormonal actions—just as a microprocessing chip controls most personal computers.

Evolution was apparently well pleased with this hormonal system—insulin, glucagon, and the eicosanoids—as a way to control an organism's response to food. So well pleased, in fact, that evolution has conserved this hormonal system for hundreds of millions of years, and made it standard operating equipment for an amazingly wide variety of species, including man. (This, by the way, is why humans can be injected with insulin—which is a protein—from pigs or cows and have no adverse reaction. Inject any other pig or beef protein into humans, and the result will be severe anaphylactic shock.)

Without food, there is no possibility of life. And without some biological system to control how the body uses food, there's no life either. That's where these hormones come in.

Insulin responses evolved to cope with the uncertainty of the food supply under extreme, potentially faminelike conditions. If animals or humans are forced to go long periods between meals (as is often the case when food comes from hunting or gathering), then the ability to store nutrients can make the difference between life and death.

When times are leaner—between meals, for example, or during fasts—declining insulin levels mean a corresponding increase in levels of glucagon. This, in turn, tells the liver to release stored carbohydrates in a controlled, measured way so as to keep the brain fed and maintain adequate mental function.

Eicosanoids, in addition to regulating insulin and glucagon, are also a primary control for the release of stored body fat, which, when liver glycogen stores are used up, becomes a backup fuel source for the brain. In addition, the release of stored body fat is your safety net during famine. Just as a runner could potentially finish twenty marathons using only stored body fat as fuel, you could live for about forty days without eating, on your stored body fat alone.

By the time mammals emerged—about forty million years ago—these systems were firmly in place. And it's a good thing too, because when man came along, with his carbohydrate-gluttonous big brain, he needed a very sophisticated and effective system to keep that hoggish brain supplied with fuel.

Bottom line: by the time man came along, all these control systems were deeply embedded in his genes. Now, genetic changes evolve very slowly. For example, the genes of humans and chimpanzees differ by less than 1 percent, even though five million years have passed since the two species diverged. Genetically, there's virtually no difference between you and your ancestors who walked the earth 100,000 years ago. In fact, mankind's genes have not changed substantially for the past one million years.

Just as evolution is a slow process, dietary patterns also change very slowly. This means that a species tends to develop a favorite menu of food types that supply it with energy, and it tends not to react very well to changes in that menu.

One hundred thousand years ago, during the Neo-Paleolithic era, herds of animals wandered about, with *Homo sapiens* following right behind. Neo-Paleolithic man was a prolific hunter, actually reducing many species to near extinction. In locales where hunting was good, people stopped to gather fruits and fiber-rich vegetables. So lean meat, fruits, and vegetables were the preferred menu—a menu in harmony with human genetic makeup.

The evidence suggests that in Neo-Paleolithic times both men and women had the bone structures of world-class athletes. What type of athletes? Definitely not long-distance runners, but more like decathletes, combining both speed and strength.

Modern analysis of Neo-Paleolithic diets makes it apparent why our ancestors were so physically developed. First of all, their carbohydrate sources—fruits and fiber-rich vegetables—were exceptionally rich in micronutrients (vitamins and minerals). In fact, it's been estimated recently that the typical diet of Neo-Paleolithic man supplied two to five times the RDA of vitamins and minerals.

Far more important, though—and this was reported in a 1985 article in the *New England Journal of Medicine*—is the fact that almost to the percentage point *Neo-Paleolithic diets have the same protein-to-carbohydrate ratio as a Zone-favorable diet.* So the Neo-Paleolithic diet kept insulin, glucagon, and eicosanoid responses on an even keel.

The question will be raised, "If Neo-Paleolithic man ate such a good Zone-favorable diet, why was his life span (approximately 18 years) so short compared to today?" The answer is that life in Neo-Paleolithic times was exceptionally harsh; humans were engaged in a constant, everyday battle with their potential dinner. Sometimes, of course, humans *became* the dinner, and that meant lots of life-shortening lethal accidents. Combine that with a high rate of killer infectious diseases, and you have a short life expectancy.

Actually, the average life expectancy did not change appreciably until after the Industrial Revolution, and much of the increase has only occurred in the last century, through better nutrition and sanitation. For example, the average life expectancy in ancient Rome (approximately twenty-two years) was not much different from that of Neo-Paleolithic man.

All this dietary and genetic harmony was disrupted about ten thousand years ago with the development of agriculture. With agriculture came two entirely new additions to the human diet: grains and dairy products.

Remember that from an evolutionary point of view ten thousand years is nothing more than the flick of an eyelash. Genomes—a species' total genetic makeup—don't change much in ten thousand years. So human genes have been adapting very reluctantly and very sluggishly to the introduction of these two new food groups ten thousand years ago. In fact, by and large *humankind has been genetically unable to cope with these foods.*

Let's first look at dairy products. All humans are born with an enzyme called lactase that allows them to break down lactose (milk sugar) in human breast milk so it can be absorbed by the body. In many people, after early childhood the activity of this enzyme decreases to very low levels, so that many adults become lactose intolerant—that is, they have trouble digesting milk and dairy products.

Only with the domestication of cattle some eight thousand years ago did cow's milk (which, like human breast milk, is rich in lactose) become widely available. The only populations which eventually evolved to retain the activity of the lactase enzyme in adulthood were those who were constantly exposed to lactose through relentless consumption of dairy products—primarily Europeans of Scandinavian descent. As a result, these people can still digest lactose as adolescents and adults.

Unfortunately, 80 percent of the world's population has not yet caught up to the Scandinavians. For the rest of the world, dairy products (unless fermented like yogurt to remove the lactose) are a digestive disaster. Maybe with another twenty thousand years of evolution, every human will be able to digest dairy products, but that's certainly not the case now.

It's essentially the same story for high-density carbohydrates like grains. You'll recall that in America approximately 25 percent of the population has a very blunted insulin response, so those people can eat high-density carbohydrates with little problem. However, there's another 25 percent of the same otherwise normal population that will have a very elevated insulin response to the intake of the same amount of high-density carbohydrates. Between those two extremes lies the rest of the American population.

Just as constant exposure to dairy products has allowed most northern Europeans to evolve genetically able to tolerate milk, I suspect that constant exposure to grain has begun to create a slow evolutionary adaptation toward reducing the typically elevated insulin response to high-density carbohydrates (like pasta). Maybe in twenty thousand years, all humans will be able to eat high-density carbohydrates without an exaggerated insulin response. Maybe then, but definitely not now.

Another consequence of the introduction of grains as a primary food ten thousand years ago was the reduced intake of low-fat animal protein. As a result, humankind actually shrank. The average height of Neo-Paleolithic man was about five feet ten, and for Neo-Paleolithic women about five feet six. Yet soon after grains were introduced into the human food chain, the average height of both men and women shrank by about six inches. It's taken ten thousand years to get that six inches back, and we actually didn't get most of it back until the twentieth century, when food in general and protein in particular became more abundant.

Unfortunately, in the process of regaining lost height, the structure of modern man came back in a different form. Instead of looking like world-class athletes, many people, at least in America, now look like Porky Pig. Why? With the increased consumption of protein has come a radically increased consumption of carbohydrates. The result: chronically elevated insulin levels, and increasing levels of body fat.

In today's supermarket, aisle after aisle displays one carbohydrate after another in different product forms. Well, the stomach can't tell the difference between a candy bar and a plate of pasta. They're both carbohydrates. If eaten to excess, they'll both cause an increase in insulin output and the accumulation of more body fat.

The problem, as I've said, is that modern man is not genetically adapted to these "civilized" foods. To be genetically correct, man needs a modern version of a Neo-Paleolithic diet, a diet that's based on his current genetic makeup. That's exactly what a Zone-favorable diet is: a diet that is synergistic with mankind's genetic structure, which has changed very little in the last 100,000 years.

So there's yet another way to think of the Zone-favorable diet: as an *evolutionary* diet. Our bodies evolved millions of years ago to eat in a particular way. We have strayed from that path, but it's simple to return by following a Zone-favorable diet, a diet that is genetically correct.

CHAPTER TEN

VITAMINS, MINERALS, AND THE ZONE

Up to this point I've been talking almost exclusively about macronutrients: protein, carbohydrate, and fat. But what about micronutrients—vitamins and minerals? Are they important? Do they have a role in a Zone-favorable diet?

A tremendous amount of the current research on nutrition has been focused on micronutrients. People seem to think that vitamins and minerals are some kind of magic elixir, and once you isolate that elixir and put it in a two-piece, hard-shell capsule, you've found the miracle of life. So pervasive is this thinking that nearly 50 percent of Americans now take vitamin and mineral supplements—in spite of U.S. government recommendations that all the vitamins and minerals you need can be found in the so-called "balanced" diet.

With good reason, people fear their "balanced" diet may not be so balanced after all. This lack of balance may be the reason they're tired, overweight, or downright ill. This fear has helped create a $3-billion-a-year industry that takes vitamins and minerals and puts them in capsules or tablets. Perhaps it's not surprising that the production of vitamins (which are really specialty chemicals) is dominated by three companies: Hoffmann-LaRoche, Pfizer, and Eastman Kodak—some of the largest drug and chemical companies in the world.

With all this money and power involved in the research and production of micronutrients, you'd think they'd be crucial in preventing disease. That's certainly what the vitamin industry and the drug companies would like you to believe, especially about the antioxidant vitamins C, E, and beta carotene.

But the truth is that many of the clinical studies using high doses of these antioxidant vitamins have produced mixed results. For example: in one recent study with 29,000 male smokers in Finland, those who received high doses of beta carotene for six years had an 18 percent greater incidence of lung cancer. In the same study, those given large doses of Vitamin E suffered an increased incidence of stroke. Another recent study showed that beta carotene, Vitamin E, and Vitamin C did not prevent precancerous lesions in the colon from subsequently developing into colon cancer.

At the same time, some studies supposedly showcasing the benefits of antioxidants may be getting the right results, but for the wrong reasons. Early studies suggested that diets rich in leafy green vegetables and fruits were protective against cancer. The fact that the sources of favorable carbohydrates in those diets were also rich in antioxidants led researchers to jump to the conclusion that it was the antioxidants protecting people from cancer.

But wait a minute: aren't green leafy vegetables and fruits the major carbohydrate components of a Zone-favorable diet? Yes, they are. So maybe the anticancer benefits in this study came not from the antioxidants, but from the fact that the subjects were eating more favorable carbohydrates. They were inadvertently following a diet that approximated a Zone-favorable diet.

Of course, there is an impressive body of results that shows positive benefits of supplementation with antioxidants. I said the data are mixed—some good, some bad, most inconclusive. Which is to say that isolated antioxidants are not magic pills. Given the choice of taking an antioxidant pill to prevent cancer or maintaining a Zone-favorable diet to limit the overproduction of bad eicosanoids that facilitate the spread of cancer (see Chapter 14), I would personally opt for the diet. I hope you would too.

This is not to say that micronutrients are not important. They are. Certain micronutrients play an important role in a Zone-favorable diet because they have an indirect effect on eicosanoids. Remember, controlling eicosanoids is what the Zone is all about. The micronutrients that affect eicosanoids fall into two classes: antioxidants and enzymatic cofactors (see Figure 10-1). To understand how they help you get to the Zone, we have to talk a little about what they actually do.

ANTIOXIDANTS

By now, almost everyone has heard of the antioxidant vitamins: vitamin E, vitamin C, and beta carotene. These particular micronutrients

**Micronutrients Important for
Successful Eicosanoid Modulation**

Antioxidants

Vitamin E

Vitamin C

Beta carotene

Co-factors

Vitamin B$_3$

Vitamin B$_6$

Zinc

Magnesium

Figure 10-1

are ballyhooed in the media as your personal shield against the attack of the dreaded free radical. What is a free radical? Technically, it's just an oxygen molecule with an electron missing (i.e., an "unpaired" electron). Ironically—and this is something the media never tells you—you need free radicals to sustain life. In fact, the life-producing effect of oxygen is only possible if oxygen is converted into free radicals. Free radicals are also some of the most important weapons in the immune system, helping to fight disease-causing bacterial invaders. Here's the kicker: without free radicals it would be impossible for the body to produce eicosanoids in the first place.

It's only when these life-sustaining free radicals hang around too long, or your body produces too many, that they begin to cause trouble. Then they're like an unwanted house guest or dead fish after three days—they wear out their welcome quickly. In fact, an over-abundance of free radicals has been implicated as a factor in causing heart disease, cancer, and a number of other troublesome ailments.

Why is this true? Because the most likely biological targets for excess free radicals are the building blocks of eicosanoids: the *essential fatty acids*, because they contain a very high level of polyunsaturation that provides a tempting target for excess free radicals to extract extra electrons. Unfortunately, in the process the essential fatty acid becomes oxidized. Essentially, these building blocks for eicosanoids are waving a molecular red flag that says "oxidize me." And once an essential fatty is oxidized, it can't be made into an eicosanoid.

That's why it's important to quench any excess production of free radicals by using antioxidants. Antioxidants are like good soldiers: they destroy free radicals by letting themselves be destroyed in the process—the ultimate sacrifice. Since antioxidants are continually being destroyed, they have to be continually replaced. So if you replace the antioxidant vitamins—vitamin E, vitamin C, and beta carotene—and maintain them at adequate levels, you'll protect the essential fatty acids so that they can be made into eicosanoids.

But what happens if you have too *many* antioxidants in the system? You guessed it: eicosanoid formation begins to slow down. (Remember, eicosanoids need free radicals to form in the first place.) So once again it's a matter of balance: too few antioxidants or too many, and the vital production of eicosanoids suffers.

The key, then, is getting adequate levels of antioxidants. What is adequate? The current Recommended Daily Allowance established by the government is 30 IU for Vitamin E, 60 mg for Vitamin C, and 5,000 IU (3 mg) for beta carotene. Current research indicates that truly adequate amounts are greater than the RDA. With that research in mind, I personally feel comfortable in recommending that you try to maintain a daily intake of 200 IU of Vitamin E, 500 mg of Vitamin C, and 10,000 IU (6 mg) of beta carotene—assuming you're following a Zone-favorable diet. These are not megadoses, but they are more than the amounts recommended by the government as the minimum to prevent deficiencies.

Where can you get these levels of antioxidants? In most cases, you don't need pills or other supplements. All you have to do is eat Zone-favorable carbohydrates.

Take a look at Table 10-1. This table shows that the levels of Vitamin C and beta carotene that I feel are beneficial are easily obtainable simply by following a Zone-favorable diet.

The one antioxidant that's hard to get in sufficient quantities without supplementation is Vitamin E. The richest dietary sources of Vitamin E consist of isolated vegetable oils—the Vitamin E con-

TABLE 10-1

Zone-favorable Sources of Vitamin C and Beta Carotene

Vitamin C (Zone-favorable recommendation is 500 mg a day, RDA is 60 mg)

Red bell peppers (1 cup)	190 mg
Honeydew melon (½)	172 mg
Broccoli (1 cup)	120 mg
Green bell peppers (1 cup)	90 mg
Strawberries (1 cup)	82 mg
Orange (1)	80 mg
Cantaloupe (½)	75 mg
Kiwi (1)	75 mg
Cauliflower (1 cup)	56 mg
Tomato (1)	24 mg
Blueberries (1 cup)	20 mg

Beta carotene (Zone-favorable recommendation is 6 mg a day, RDA is 3 mg)

Spinach (1 cup cooked)	9.8 mg
Cantaloupe (½)	4.8 mg
Apricots (2)	2.5 mg
Romaine lettuce (1 cup)	1.1 mg

tained in the oil seed is there to protect the polyunsaturated essential fatty acids from oxidation. Since a Zone-favorable diet is also a low-total-fat diet, getting adequate Vitamin E might be a problem. So this is one of the few instances in which I would recommend supplementation, but with 200 IU of Vitamin E per day as a recommended level.

ENZYMATIC COFACTORS

The other group of important micronutrients are the enzymatic cofactors, including vitamin B_6, vitamin B_3, magnesium, and zinc. These enzymatic cofactors are required for both essential fatty acid metabolism and eicosanoid formation.

Even if the essential fatty acids have been protected with adequate levels of antioxidants, they still must be transformed into eicosanoids. That's where the enzymatic cofactors come in. Without them, the whole process of eicosanoid formation will be severely limited. Again, you don't need megadoses of these micronutrients, but they must be part of your diet.

What are the richest sources of these enzymatic cofactors? By now it should be no surprise: the richest sources are also the primary components of a Zone-favorable diet (see Table 10-2).

As you can see, most of the foods rich in the key enzymatic cofactors are Zone-favorable, low-fat protein sources. Unfavorable carbohydrates, which you should be using in moderation anyway, are a relatively poor source of these essential enzymatic cofactors. Just another reason to follow a Zone-favorable diet.

As I said earlier, all these micronutrients—antioxidants and enzymatic cofactors—are important as role players for eicosanoid formation. So in a way it's not surprising that these vitamins and minerals are the same ones that have been elevated to icon status by the health-food industry.

We're always hearing about Aunt Millie, who takes vitamin B_6 for her arthritis. Or Uncle Bob, who takes vitamin C to cure cancer. Or Cousin Jim, who takes vitamin E to treat his bad heart. In each of those conditions, there's a common link. Each of these disease states can be viewed as a consequence of a long-term overproduction of bad eicosanoids. So it may have been that supplementation with those micronutrients was just enough to produce a favorable balance of eicosanoids for Aunt Millie, Uncle Bob, or Cousin Jim.

But the real benefits may have come from the fact that their diets were *almost* Zone-favorable. So the diet itself may have gotten them closer to the Zone, and the extra micronutrients were enough to actually push them into the Zone, where it's easier to treat and even cure diseases.

What might have worked for Aunt Millie and Uncle Bob may not (and probably will not) work for the vast majority of people. Yes, micronutrients are important, but in the story of the Zone they remain secondary players. If you plan to get to the Zone, then controlling the balance of macronutrients in your diet will be ten to one hundred times more important than the amount of micronutrients you consume. Besides, you should be getting all the micronu-

TABLE 10-2

Zone-favorable Sources of Enzymatic Cofactors

	PERCENTAGE RDA

Vitamin B₃

Tuna (4 oz.)	65%
Turkey (4 oz.)	55%
Chicken (4 oz.)	55%
Salmon (4 oz.)	37%

Vitamin B₆

Tuna (4 oz.)	45%
Salmon (4 oz.)	35%
Trout (4 oz.)	35%
Turkey (4 oz.)	27%
Chicken (4 oz.)	27%

Zinc

Cod (4 oz.)	97%
Kidney beans (4 oz.)	29%
Turkey (4 oz.)	23%

Magnesium

Tuna (4 oz.)	42%
Tofu (6 oz.)	33%
Sole (4 oz.)	18%

trients you need (except vitamin E) just by following a Zone-favorable diet.

Is taking extra micronutrients a bad idea? Of course not. In fact, as long as you do it in moderation, it can be a relatively inexpensive insurance policy. But if you consume large amounts of micronutrients, and don't eat a Zone-favorable diet, you haven't done anything of consequence to help you reach the Zone. You're probably spitting in the wind. Supplementing your diet with micronutrients without simultaneously controlling the macronutrient balance is like building

a sand castle on the beach to protect yourself from an oncoming hormonal tidal wave.

If you want to help treat and prevent the likelihood of disease,
think about reaching the Zone through your diet—instead of reaching for some magic vitamin pill.

CHAPTER ELEVEN

ASPIRIN: THE WONDER DRUG

Of all the wonder drugs this century has produced, aspirin may well be the most important. No other drug has such sweeping effects. It fights pain, controls fever, reduces inflammation, and helps prevent heart attacks and strokes. Preliminary indications are that it may also help prevent cancer. For such a commonplace drug, aspirin is amazingly versatile.

Yet for the first seventy years after its introduction by the German drug manufacturing company Farbenfabriken Bayer, no one knew how aspirin really worked. In fact, as recently as 1966, the *New York Times Magazine* called aspirin "The Wonder Drug Nobody Understands."

The breakthrough in explaining the mechanics of aspirin came in the late 1960s, when John Vane, a pharmacologist at the Royal College of Surgeons in London, England, discovered that aspirin stopped the body's cells from manufacturing an important subclass of eicosanoids called *prostaglandins.* How does aspirin accomplish this task? It conducts a suicide mission to destroy a single *cyclooxygenase enzyme*, the key enzyme that controls the production of all prostaglandins.

One molecule of aspirin, it turns out, will totally destroy one cyclooxygenase enzyme. It takes about four to six hours for the body to make more of the enzyme, so depending on how much aspirin is taken your body is making very few prostaglandins, good or bad.

Aspirin's impact on prostaglandin formation turns out to be the key to all of its wide-ranging effects. Like aspirin itself, many prostaglandins are biological jacks-of-all-trades: they help regulate the widening and narrowing of blood vessels and the onset of inflammation, especially in the joints. The discovery that aspirin put the brakes on the manufacture of certain bad eicosanoids explained its role in combating pain, fever, and inflammation, and set the foundation for understanding its importance in preventing heart attack, stroke, and cancer.

In 1982, Vane's earlier discovery won him a portion of the most coveted of all scientific honors: the Nobel Prize in Medicine. But he still hadn't explained aspirin's role in preventing blood clotting—the secret of its success in preventing heart attacks and strokes. In the mid-1970s a team led by Swedish researcher Bengt Samuelsson of the Karolinska Institute in Stockholm discovered that one of the prostaglandins, known as prostaglandin G_2, could be transformed into yet another eicosanoid called thromboxane A_2 (see Figure 11-1). That discovery gave Samuelsson a share of the 1982 Nobel Prize in Medicine. (The third recipient was Sune Bergstrom, also from the Karolinska Institute, for his unraveling of the structure of eicosanoids.)

Thromboxane A_2, Samuelsson found, caused blood platelets to clump together and form clots. If the clots grew big enough, they could clog the blood vessels, leading to heart attacks or strokes. Vane's discovery of aspirin's mode of action now explained why it also stopped the manufacture of thromboxane A_2: by preventing the formation of the prostaglandin that was thromboxane's biological "parent." Aspirin limited the formation of life-threatening blood clots.

(Given its role in setting the stage for heart attacks, it's not surprising that thromboxane A_2 is considered one of the most dangerous of the bad eicosanoids. But in reality some thromboxane A_2 is always needed. Without it, we would bleed to death from even minor cuts. Again, we see the necessity of maintaining a balance of good and bad eicosanoids.)

Samuelsson had explained the mechanism by which aspirin might prevent heart attacks. But the research that elevated aspirin to the world spotlight wasn't reported until 1988, when the *New England Journal of Medicine* announced the results of a study showing that aspirin decreased the number of heart attacks in healthy male physicians by 40 percent. Virtually overnight, aspirin became the most inexpensive drug in history to prevent heart attacks.

(Although Samuelsson and the *New England Journal* researchers got the praise—and the prizes—for discovering the benefits of aspirin in heart-attack prevention, those benefits had actually been reported more than thirty years earlier by a lonely pioneer in cardiovascular treatment, Dr. Lawrence Craven. Unfortunately, he published his findings in the obscure *Mississippi Valley Medical Journal*. Had Dr.

**Arachidonic-Acid Metabolism via
Cyclooxygenase Enzyme**

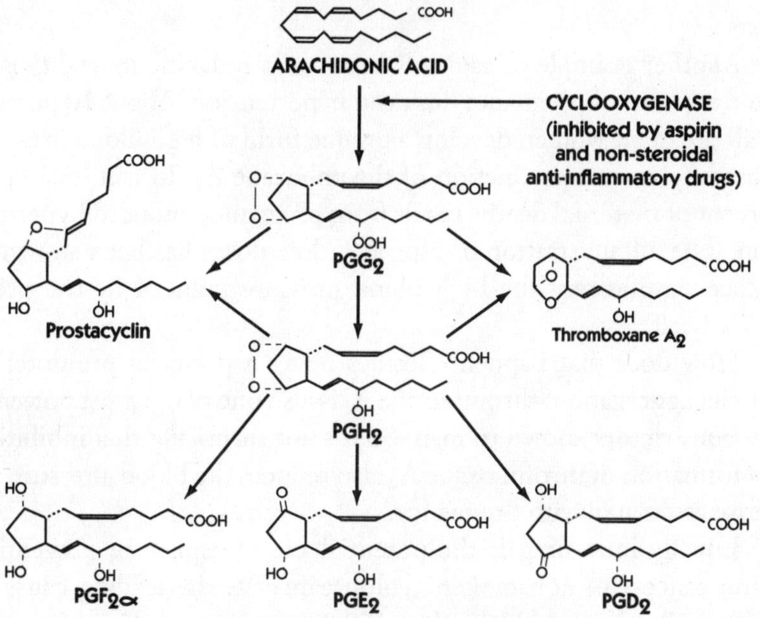

Figure 11-1

Craven picked a slightly more prestigious and therefore more quotable journal, who knows how many millions of heart attacks might have been prevented? Perhaps even the premature deaths of my father and his brothers.)

In terms of revealing the lifesaving potential of aspirin, these studies were truly monumental. Let's look at the numbers. Based on preliminary research, aspirin can potentially produce nearly a 40 percent reduction in the incidence of heart attacks, and possibly a 20 percent reduction in strokes. These are not insignificant numbers—1,500,000 heart attacks occur each year, killing more than 500,000 people. At the same time, 400,000 people are victimized by strokes each year, and more than 100,000 of these stroke victims die.

It takes only the simplest of mathematics to show that the proper use of aspirin could potentially prevent more than 600,000 heart attacks per year, saving more than 200,000 lives. Similarly, as many as 80,000 strokes could potentially be prevented, saving nearly 20,000 lives annually. This saving in lives is equivalent to eliminating over-night the annual deaths caused by lung cancer, the most common form of cancer. It would also save billions of dollars in health-care costs.

Another example of aspirin's benefits in reducing mortality is in the treatment of pregnancy-induced hypertension. About 10 percent of all pregnant women develop a unique form of high blood pressure caused by an overproduction of thromboxane A_2. In fact, nearly 20 percent of maternal deaths result from pregnancy-induced hypertension. The administration of aspirin in low doses has been shown to reduce significantly the high blood pressure induced by the pregnancy itself.

How does that happen? Besides being a powerful promoter of platelet aggregation, thromboxane A_2 is also one of the most powerful vasoconstrictors known to man. So it's not surprising that inhibiting the formation of thromboxane A_2 also reduces the blood-pressure increase associated with pregnancy.

Equally intriguing is the potential use of aspirin in preventing colon cancer. In nonsmokers, colon cancer is the leading cause of cancer-related death. More than 150,000 people develop colon cancer every year, and more than one-third of these patients die of the disease. In fact, the number of annual deaths from colon cancer (58,-000) is far greater than the number of deaths from breast cancer (46,-000). A 1991 study reported in the *New England Journal of Medicine* showed that regular aspirin use could reduce colon-cancer death rates in both men and women by more than 40 percent.

Like heart disease, cancer can be viewed as resulting from an on-going imbalance of eicosanoids. Immune-system cells known as natural killer (NK) cells are one of the primary natural defenses against cancer. In effect, NK cells are the body's cancer police, always searching for abnormal cells to destroy. But the activity of NK cells is decreased by bad eicosanoids like PGE_2. Obviously, if the activity of NK cells is decreased, cancer cells will have a far better chance for survival and eventual growth.

Remember that aspirin is a nonselective inhibitor of prostaglandin production. So, as it knocks out PGE_2 to reduce inflammation and pain, it simultaneously reduces the same prostaglandin that knocks out NK cells. The end result: the body's own defense system is now more likely to detect and destroy abnormal cancer cells before they form life-threatening tumors.

Although the effects of aspirin on heart attacks and pregnancy-induced hypertension—as well as its potential effect as a cancer fighter—are nothing short of spectacular, its most common use is still to treat the simpler ills of mankind, such as headaches and fevers. Here another fascinating aspect of the role that eicosanoids play in the body becomes apparent.

The pain of a headache can come either from constriction of the blood vessels to the brain, or simply from the excess release of the body's "pain chemicals"—bad eicosanoids. Sometimes both events occur simultaneously.

Aspirin takes care of both of them. As we've already seen, it reduces vasoconstriction by reducing levels of thromboxane A_2. But how about pain? Again, PGE_2 is a key player. PGE_2 is the principal mediator of both pain and fever. When aspirin inhibits the formation of all prostaglandins, it also shuts down production of PGE_2. Once PGE_2 production is inhibited, pain and fever are also reduced. So the wonder drug is working its wonders simply by temporarily shutting down the overproduction of bad eicosanoids.

Heart disease, cancer, hypertension, pain, and fever—the list of maladies that can be treated, if not actually prevented, with aspirin is long and impressive. But aspirin also has a dark side—in fact, it's far from a totally safe drug. Aspirin's side effects are significant and they can be quite ugly.

Let's take the case of pregnancy. Even though aspirin reduces pregnancy-induced hypertension, it can also induce abortion and internal bleeding. So prescribing aspirin to reduce pregnancy-induced hypertension must be carefully balanced by a doctor. (Because of the danger of bleeding, the same caution should be exercised by the millions of Americans taking aspirin for the relief of chronic arthritis pain.)

In addition, every year there are more than ten thousand reported cases of aspirin overdose for a wide variety of reasons. Few people know it, but at high enough levels aspirin can cause death. It's not a totally innocuous drug, even though you can find it in every supermarket—often right alongside the bagels.

The truth is that aspirin is not a very sophisticated drug. It's like a medicinal sledgehammer: when it knocks out bad prostaglandins, it simultaneously knocks out good prostaglandins. If you're producing an overabundance of bad prostaglandins (manifested in a headache or arthritic pain), you don't mind knocking out some good prostaglandins to get temporary relief. But if you do this on a long-term basis, prostaglandin formation is decreased throughout the body.

When this happens, platelets don't clump when they're supposed to (which can give rise to internal bleeding), bicarbonate in the stomach isn't secreted (ulcers can develop), and gastrointestinal (GI) tract bleeding can take place. (Ironically, the newest breakthrough drug to prevent aspirin-induced GI bleeding is a synthetic version of a good eicosanoid, PGE_1, called misoprostol.) Potentially even worse, long-term use of aspirin can eventually depress the immune system. There are other problems. For example, it's possible to develop a sensitivity to aspirin. When the formation of prostaglandins is inhibited, arachidonic acid in the body doesn't simply disappear. It gets diverted to another subclass of eicosanoids called *leukotrienes*, which are the mediators of allergies. So people can ultimately become allergic to the very drug that's supposed to be curing them.

Aspirin is a two-edged sword. It can treat or prevent illness, but it can also make people sick. What we need is a drug that has all of aspirin's benefits without any of its side effects. A more sophisticated drug would increase levels of good eicosanoids while simultaneously decreasing the bad eicosanoids, and not have any side effects.

What is that drug? Food, when you're following a Zone-favorable diet.

Remember that aspirin is only doing a crude job of modulating only one subgroup of eicosanoids (prostaglandins) by knocking out all of them—good and bad. But following a Zone-favorable diet will maintain an appropriate and healthful balance of good and bad eicosanoids, stimulating the production of the right amount of good eicosanoids, knocking out the right amount of bad ones, and doing it with a precision that aspirin can never approximate.

If aspirin is a wonder drug, then eicosanoids are the wonder hormones.

CHAPTER TWELVE

THE WONDER HORMONES: EICOSANOIDS—THE LONG COURSE

Remember the last time you had the flu? If you're like me, you probably took a couple of aspirins. Although the aspirins didn't cure the disease, within a few minutes after taking them you started to feel better. The flu symptoms seemed to abate, your fever went down, and your head felt clearer, your mind sharper.

Why did aspirin have such a dramatic impact on how you felt? As you've learned, it's because aspirin acts on the prostaglandins—that important subgroup of the eicosanoid family.

In fact, without the discovery of the connection between aspirin and prostaglandins, I would not be writing this book. That discovery, and its profound implications for treating and preventing heart disease, started me on the highway toward understanding the Zone.

In the last chapter I outlined some of the reasons why aspirin has such powerful benefits. But can aspirin get you to the Zone? No.

Aspirin does temporarily alter the balance of good and bad eicosanoids by shutting down the production of all prostaglandins, so it affects the Zone in a crude way. If you're making too many bad eicosanoids, aspirin will tilt the balance in your favor for a short time. But your goal is to keep that balance in your favor constantly. That can only be done with food.

To understand in greater detail the crucial link between diet and the Zone, you should be familiar with the important nutritional code that determines what type of eicosanoids (good or bad) the body makes in the first place. In many ways this nutritional code is just as important as your genetic code. The more you understand it, the better you'll be prepared to stay in the Zone on a constant basis.

One feature of this nutritional code is that it challenges many of

the current assumptions concerning the role of dietary fat. In many
ways fat is the central character in the story of the Zone. Remember,
the eventual production of all eicosanoids uses as its basic raw mate-
rial a group of fat substances known as essential fatty acids. These
fatty acids must be supplied by fat in the diet. They can't be made by
the body.

There are a total of eight essential fatty acids, which fall into two
classes—omega 6 and omega 3 fatty acids. Although both classes can
be made into eicosanoids, omega 6 fatty acids are the most important
for reaching the Zone. The eicosanoids that come from omega 3 fatty
acids are relatively neutral. They don't do much one way or the other.
However, omega 6 fatty acids are the building blocks for both good
and bad eicosanoids. To boil it down, *the effect of diet (particularly the*

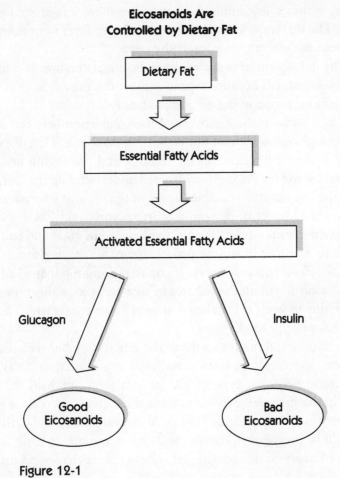

**Eicosanoids Are
Controlled by Dietary Fat**

Figure 12-1

protein-to-carbohydrate ratio of the meals you eat) on the metabolic fate of omega 6 fatty acids determines whether or not you will ever enter the Zone.

The production of good or bad eicosanoids begins with the baby of the omega 6 family: an essential fatty acid known as *linoleic acid.* (I call it the "baby" because linoleic acid cannot be made into an eicosanoid until it is further metabolized into substances that are the true building blocks of eicosanoids.) Linoleic acid is found in virtually every food—protein, vegetables, even grains. In most cases, the higher the fat content of a food, the higher the linoleic acid content.

If linoleic acid is the baby, then the molecular "strollers" that actually carry linoleic acid to the cells are low-density lipoproteins (LDL—the same substances that carry bad cholesterol). Without LDL's constantly delivering linoleic acid to the cells, there would be no way for a cell to make an eicosanoid. (Here's another example of a supposedly "bad" substance doing a good job.)

Since linoleic acid is essentially a helpless infant, once it reaches the cells it needs to do a lot of "growing" before it can be made into an eicosanoid. That "growth" is actually a cascade of transformations—molecular events that can be viewed as the stages of development in linoleic acid's conversion into an "adult" eicosanoid.

The first step in this conversion process takes place when a key enzyme called *delta 6 desaturase* converts the linoleic acid to a more metabolically activated fatty acid known as *gamma linolenic acid* (GLA). (You might think of this as the "baby" reaching "adolescence" with the help of an influential "teacher"—delta 6 desaturase.) Unlike linoleic acid, which is found in virtually every food, GLA is rarely found in food. In fact, the richest source of GLA is human breast milk, although trace amounts can be found in one other common food—oatmeal.

GLA is considered an "activated" essential fatty acid because very small amounts fill the metabolic pipelines that allow the body to make other activated essential fatty acids. This is shown in Figure 12-1. If for some reason the body is not making enough activated essential fatty acids such as GLA, there is no way to make enough eicosanoids (good or bad), and no way to optimize body function.

In other words, if you ever want to get to the Zone, your body's omega 6 metabolic pipeline must be filled with an adequate amount of GLA.

There are two times in life when the body's ability to produce

GLA from linoleic acid is compromised, thus creating a potentially significant disruption of eicosanoid production—both good and bad. The first time is at birth. It takes about six months after birth before the delta 6 desaturase enzyme reaches full activity. During this period the essential supplies of GLA (which the infant still can't make effectively) comes only from mother's breast milk.

This explains why breast-fed babies invariably are healthier and leaner than bottle-fed babies. They have a higher dietary intake of GLA, and therefore can make more good eicosanoids. On the other hand, the cow's milk and/or soy milk used in infant formulas contain virtually no GLA. (Nestlé, a leading infant-formula manufacturer and food-processing giant, has mounted a major research program over the last ten years to isolate GLA and incorporate it into infant formulas.)

Six months after birth, when the delta 6 desaturase enzyme comes to full activity (you might think of this as the "teacher" getting "certified"), babies can be weaned from breast milk, because they can now use dietary linoleic acid to make adequate levels of GLA on their own.

The second time that the body's ability to make GLA is compromised is after the age of thirty. As people age, the activity of the delta 6 desaturase enzyme slows down. Scientific studies have indicated that the ability to make eicosanoids at age sixty-five is one-third what it was at age twenty-five.

Furthermore, many of the chronic diseases associated with aging—heart disease, arthritis, and cancer, for example—are strongly connected with eicosanoid imbalances (if not actual deficiencies). These may result from the slowdown in delta 6 desaturase activity. As we age, it becomes more and more difficult to reach the Zone. But one of the most important benefits of a Zone-favorable diet is that it speeds up the natural activity of the delta 6 desaturase enzyme even as you age. So in essence, if you follow these dietary guidelines, you're generating youthful levels of GLA even though you're getting older.

Are there other factors besides aging that can decrease the body's ability to make GLA? Yes. Some are listed in Figure 12-2. We've already seen the effects of aging, so now let's look at the others.

Of all the factors that influence GLA production, perhaps the most important—and certainly the most manageable—is diet. There are three ways that diet can adversely affect the activity of delta 6

**Factors That Can Depress
Delta 6 Desaturase Activity**

Aging

Diet
Alpha linolenic acid, Trans fatty acids

Disease
Viral infections

Stress-Related Hormones
Cortisol, Adrenaline

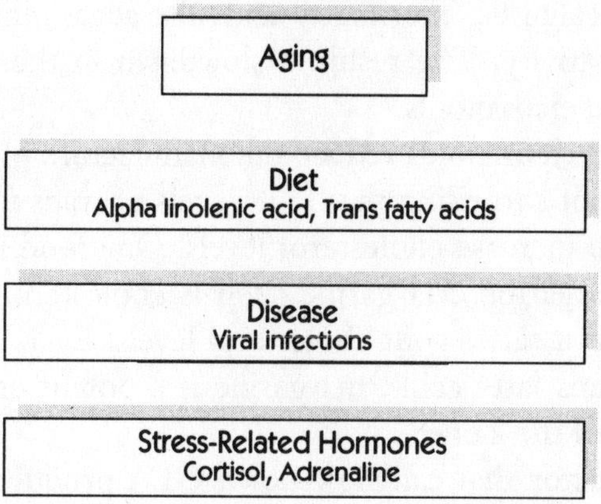

Figure 12-2

desaturase, thereby decreasing GLA production. The surest way is to eat a high carbohydrate diet. High levels of carbohydrates in the bloodstream will slow down delta 6 desaturase activity and decrease GLA production. Decrease GLA production, and you'll limit the production of good eicosanoids. Limit good eicosanoid production, and you're more likely to get fatter and less healthy—just like the bottle-fed child compared to the breast-fed child.

High-carb diets have an obvious effect on delta 6 desaturase. But there are more insidious ways to further reduce the production of this crucial enzyme, and thus limit the formation of GLA. One is to consume large amounts of alpha linolenic acid (ALA). This is an omega 3 fatty acid that's found in high amounts in flax seeds, flax seed oil, and walnuts.

ALA is like a wet blanket for the enzymes that control the eventual flow of omega 6 essential fatty acids toward eicosanoids. In many ways ALA is the biological equivalent of aspirin: by limiting the activity of the delta 6 desaturase enzyme, it knocks out the production of both good and bad eicosanoids.

Another man-made dietary invention also has very adverse consequences for eicosanoid production. This is the development of partially hydrogenated vegetable oils that contain trans fatty acids. These artificially produced oils are less likely to go rancid, so they are widely used in the food industry. Although foods containing trans fatty acids are less likely to spoil, consumers of these foods pay a severe biochemical price. Trans fatty acids also act as inhibitors of delta 6 desaturase activity. The result: a slowdown in the production of GLA and good eicosanoids.

Since good eicosanoids reduce the manufacture of cholesterol in the liver, it's not surprising that high levels of trans fatty acids have been shown to increase cholesterol levels. One food is rich in trans fatty acids: margarine. Margarine itself is cholesterol free, but that doesn't matter: it raises your cholesterol levels. Even worse, because it's high in trans fatty acids, margarine is a potent enemy that will drive you out of the Zone.

Another factor that can slow down GLA production is disease, especially viral disease. Studies conducted at Ohio State University have shown that in patients with long-term chronic fatigue after Epstein-Barr virus infection, the activity of the delta 6 desaturase enzyme remains depressed. This effectively shuts down the pipeline for good eicosanoid production.

It may well be that chronic fatigue is simply a result of an underproduction of GLA (I'll talk about this in a later chapter). It's also likely that all viral infections—from the common cold to HIV—may have similar effects on GLA formation, but to varying degrees, depending on the virulence of the virus. But if you do get a virus, having an adequate amount of GLA in your cells can help fight it off.

The final influence on GLA formation is stress. In an increasingly complex society, stress is a constant companion. It has a dramatic impact on us emotionally and physically. The body reacts to stress by producing elevated blood levels of the hormones adrenaline and cortisol. Elevated adrenaline decreases the activity of the enzyme that makes GLA, and that in turn decreases the production of good eicosanoids. Cortisol increases insulin levels, leading to an overproduction of bad eicosanoids. So stress is like a one-two punch. It does a great job of keeping you away from the Zone.

Of the major factors influencing the production of GLA (diet, viral infections, and stress), diet is the most firmly under your control. You can easily modify each of the three dietary factors I just mentioned to ensure that you're not closing down the metabolic factories that produce GLA. It's not hard to reduce excessive amounts of carbohydrate in the foods you eat, and it's not hard to avoid eating excessive amounts of ALA or trans fatty acids. You can accomplish all three simply by following a Zone-favorable diet.

To sum up: maintaining adequate levels of GLA is critically important for optimal health. The best way to ensure adequate levels of GLA is to watch the type of fat you eat, and follow a Zone-favorable diet.

Even so, filling the activated essential fatty-acid pipeline with GLA is only the first step in your journey toward reaching the Zone. To fully play its part in the production of eicosanoids, GLA must be converted to another fatty acid, called *dihomo gamma linolenic acid* (DGLA). This conversion is a relatively rapid process. If you have adequate levels of GLA in your body, this next part of the journey toward the Zone is guaranteed. On the other hand, if your levels of GLA are low, the conversion of GLA to DGLA is compromised, and so is your likelihood of reaching the Zone.

It's only with DGLA that the production of good and bad eicosanoids begins in earnest. At this point, the eicosanoid flow separates into two branches. In one branch, DGLA becomes the building block of good eicosanoids like PGE_1. In the other branch, DGLA is converted by another enzyme—called *delta 5 desaturase*—into yet another activated essential fatty acid: *arachidonic acid*.

In essence, delta 5 desaturase acts like a valve in an irrigation project by directing the flow of activated essential fatty acids. It leaves some of the DGLA to be made into good eicosanoids, and it diverts some of the DGLA to form arachidonic acid, which then triggers the manufacture of bad eicosanoids. (This is shown in Figure 12-3.)

Excess arachidonic acid is your worst biological nightmare. It's the building block for bad eicosanoids, including thromboxane A_2 (which causes platelet clumping), PGE_2 (which promotes pain and depresses the immune system) and leukotrienes (which promote allergies and skin disorders). In fact, arachidonic acid is so potent and so dangerous that when you inject it into the bloodstream of rabbits the animals die within three minutes.

The balance of DGLA to arachidonic acid in every cell in the body determines whether or not good or bad eicosanoids are made when that cell is stimulated by its external environment. The balance of DGLA to arachidonic acid is the foundation of the Zone, and it is

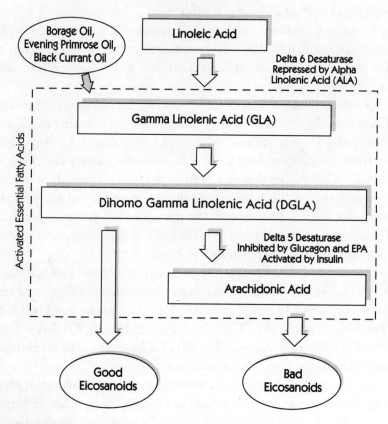

Figure 12-3

entirely controlled by the activity of this single enzyme—delta 5 desaturase.

The more active the delta 5 desaturase enzyme, the greater the potential for manufacturing more arachidonic acid. The less active the enzyme, the greater the manufacture of DGLA. Obviously, you want your body to make more DGLA and less arachidonic acid, so that it can make more good eicosanoids and fewer bad ones.

What controls the activity of delta 5 desaturase? Hormones—specifically, insulin and glucagon. Delta 5 desaturase is activated by insulin and inhibited by glucagon. So at the molecular level it's the dynamic balance of insulin and glucagon (controlled by a Zone-favorable diet) that allows you to regulate this enzymatic valve, and regulate it with a laserlike precision no drug could hope to achieve. That precision will allow you to control the building blocks for good and bad eicosanoids.

Linoleic acid, GLA, ALA, DGLA, arachidonic acid, and the delta desaturase enzymes—that's a long roster of vital players in the complex metabolic game that regulates eicosanoids. But hold on—there's one more important ingredient to add to this alphabet soup. That ingredient is another essential fatty acid, called *eicosapentaenoic acid* (EPA), a member of the omega 3 family of fatty acids. Like all omega 3 essential fatty acids, EPA is a regulator of the key enzymes that control the flow of omega 6 essential acids as they progress toward their eventual eicosanoid destination.

While EPA is a direct molecular building block for selected types of eicosanoids, these eicosanoids don't do much positively or negatively. Why is EPA so important? Because it inhibits the activity of the delta 5 desaturase enzyme that makes arachidonic acid. The payoff? Eating adequate amounts of EPA becomes another part of an overall dietary strategy to help put the clamps on the overproduction of bad eicosanoids.

Where do you find EPA? It's in some fish. The richest (and to me, the tastiest) source is salmon. Other good sources of EPA are sardines and mackerel. Low-fat fish, such as cod or flounder, contain only trace amounts of EPA.

How much fish should you eat? A 1985 study published in the *New England Journal of Medicine* indicated that 200 mg of EPA per week was enough to reduce significantly the risk of heart attack. That's one serving of salmon or three servings of tuna per week.

Why am I going into all of this detail on omega 6 fatty-acid metabolism? Because I initially thought I could access the Zone using activated essential fatty acids alone. In 1982, my thinking was that if GLA and EPA are so important in making good eicosanoids, why not simply add these activated essential fatty acids to the diet, and forget all the hassle of controlling the macronutrient content? I thought if I could supply the correct ratio of GLA and EPA in a capsule, I could control the balance of good and bad eicosanoids.

With my pharmaceutical background, I also had a "magic bullet" mentality. If I could develop a suitable magic pill composed of GLA (to fill the activated essential fatty-acid pipeline) and EPA (to reduce the activity of the delta 5 desaturase enzyme), people could eat whatever they wanted, take a few capsules containing GLA and EPA, and get to the Zone. Unfortunately, life is seldom so simple—and neither is the Zone.

In my early efforts, I thought it was only a matter of isolating enough GLA and EPA and determining the correct ratio necessary to control the balance of good and bad eicosanoids. Obviously, there was plenty of fish in the sea to provide EPA, but there was one problem with crude fish oil: it tends to be contaminated with really nasty things, like heavy metals and PCBs.

Getting rid of the heavy metals requires only a simple refining process, but the PCBs are a different matter. The only way to remove PCBs from fish oil is by a sophisticated chemical engineering process known as molecular distillation. Still, that type of chemical engineering already existed, so to make isolated EPA suitable for human consumption was an expensive but feasible process. So half the equation was in place, or so I thought.

But GLA was a different story. There are very few sources of GLA on the planet, and the best source, human breast milk, is in relatively short supply. The only other common food that contained GLA is oatmeal, but the amount of GLA in oatmeal is exceptionally small—only trace amounts.

If I were ever to find a large enough supply of GLA to make a commercial impact, I had to find some botanical source that could be grown on an industrial basis. So my brother Doug and I sat down in the bowels of the MIT library to search out seed sources rich in GLA. Of the 250,000 known seeds, only about 250 contained any GLA at all. Of the 250, only five contained any significant amounts of GLA. And of the five, only one had potential as a candidate for large-scale oil-seed production. That one botanical source was borage. (Never heard of borage? Neither had I. But it's been mentioned in the literature since the twelfth century, and today it's used primarily as an ornamental herb in English gardens.)

Okay, there wasn't a lot of it, but at least it had potential. Other potential sources, such as evening-primrose oil and black-currant oil, had significant inherent problems that limited their commercial use. (Black-currant oil had too much ALA, while evening-primrose seeds were hard to process, and the oil was very poor in GLA content.)

So in 1983 Doug and I set out to corner the world's borage market. At about the same time, the Hunt brothers were trying to corner the world market for silver. They failed, but the Sears brothers succeeded—-on the borage front, at least. Frankly, it wasn't too hard, since most of the borage seeds in the world could fit into the back seat of a car.

So in terms of borage, we owned virtually all the seeds in the world. The next step was to learn how to grow it. It turns out that borage plants grow well in only two places: the lower valleys of New Zealand and the upper plains of Saskatchewan in Canada. (This is because GLA is produced in plants as a response to low temperature—it's almost like a botanical antifreeze.) Since Saskatchewan was closer, we moved there for a year and a half to learn how to grow borage commercially, and to isolate the oil from the seeds to make it suitable for human consumption.

By 1985, we were ready to introduce borage oil into the United States for the first time. However, I knew that simply supplementing the diet with GLA was ultimately counterproductive without simultaneously supplementing it with the appropriate amount of EPA.

The question was how much EPA was needed for a given amount of GLA? Using ourselves as human guinea pigs, Doug and I found certain ratios of GLA and EPA supplements that seemed to do a pretty good job of getting us to the Zone. And, of course, we assumed that everyone in the world had the same biochemistry as we did.

Now I thought I was on my way to fame and fortune for developing the first practical dietary application of the 1982 Nobel Prize for Medicine. But this enthusiasm was quickly muted by our early work with both elite athletes and cardiovascular patients. To put it briefly, when I looked at the results of GLA and EPA supplementation in these groups, I realized that we were not consistently getting the results that we should have with this relatively crude form of eicosanoid modulation. In some cases the combination of the EPA and GLA gave spectacular results. In other cases I initially got great results, but then there was a dropoff. In still other cases, nothing happened at all.

At first I got around this problem by constantly changing the ratio of GLA to EPA for each individual. This seemed to work out somewhat better. However, it became apparent that to stay in the Zone using activated essential fatty-acid supplements alone required a constant readjustment of the ratio of GLA to EPA for each individual. So getting into the Zone using only activated essential fatty acids became an art form, not a science. Obviously I was missing a big piece of the puzzle, but what? One of the clues was the difference in results between men and women. In women, I noticed, I had to change the ratio of EPA to GLA to a much greater extent than I did for men. This sent me back to the MIT library to try to understand why.

The answer lay buried deep in some rather obscure journals. But it was a relatively simple answer: the delta 5 desaturase enzyme is under profound hormonal control. Although EPA could provide some limited control of delta 5 desaturase enzyme activity, consistent control could only be achieved by controlling hormonal balance. And which hormones? Of course: insulin and glucagon.

I finally began to understand why women seemed to need a more or less continual readjustment of the EPA to GLA ratio to stay in the Zone. Women tend to eat relatively lower amounts of protein than men, simply because more women are perpetually on low-fat, high-carbohydrate diets—which are also low in protein. As a result of these high-carbohydrate diets, the supplemented GLA was constantly being driven toward arachidonic acid because the activating effect of insulin was overwhelming the inhibitory effect of EPA.

So for women the ratio of DGLA to arachidonic acid would initially increase, and then begin to decrease as arachidonic acid built up over time. This was especially true if they were eating a high-carbohydrate diet. That's why the women constantly needed less and less GLA and more and more EPA to stay in the Zone.

At that point I realized that to get to the Zone on a consistent basis, it was far more important to control the insulin-to-glucagon ratio than it is to supplement the diet with activated essential fatty acids. That's when I shifted gears, and started to put more and more emphasis on the control of the protein-to-carbohydrate ratio as the primary portal to the Zone. With this new emphasis on the macronutrient content of the diet came a surprising discovery, a discovery applicable to both men and women. The closer a person maintained an ideal protein-to-carbohydrate ratio of 0.75, I found, the more there was a significant increase in the activity of the delta 6 desaturase enzyme.

In essence, maintaining a Zone-favorable diet prevents the normal reduction of activity of this enzyme caused by the aging process. And if the activity of the delta 6 desaturase enzyme is increased, there is little need for any extensive supplementation with GLA in the first place, since the body is now making more than sufficient levels of GLA to fill the activated essential fatty-acid pipelines.

So after cornering the borage market in 1983, I have now come to realize that as long as a normal person follows a Zone-favorable diet, that person can get all the GLA he or she needs simply by eating three to five bowls of oatmeal per week. This is because a Zone-favorable diet increases the natural production of GLA, so only small amounts of additional GLA are needed as a sort of nutritional insurance policy. So much for my sugar plum dreams of thousands of acres of borage supplying the GLA needs of the world.

At least my year and a half in Canada was interesting— fruitless, but interesting.

I tell this story only to remind you: just as in the case of vitamins and minerals, never let the tail wag the dog. Controlling the activity of the delta 5 desaturase enzyme (which is really the gateway to the Zone) is best done not by taking supplements of activated essential fatty acids, but by following a Zone-favorable diet.

Still, just as taking vitamins and minerals can provide an extra insurance policy, so can additional EPA. The best way to get EPA? Eat fish like salmon. If you don't like salmon, then try swordfish or tuna, which have lower levels of EPA. People who don't like *any* kind of fish might consider supplementation with fish-oil capsules, but make sure you buy a brand that has undergone molecular distillation to get the contaminants (like PCBs) out.

If you want to ensure that you're getting adequate GLA (which for most healthy people will be 1 to 2 mg per day), eat cooked (not instant) oatmeal three to five times a week. And if you are adding GLA supplements to your diet, always add at least fifty to a hundred times more EPA—those are the proportions of GLA and EPA you'll need to stay in the Zone.

But remember: the best amount of supplementation is always the least amount, and the best source of activated essential fatty acids is always food.

BENEFITS OF A FAVORABLE BALANCE OF
DGLA TO ARACHIDONIC ACID

If you can keep the ratio of DGLA to arachidonic acid in the appropriate balance, what biological rewards will you reap? Since many of the drugs (aspirin, nonsteroidal anti-inflammatories [NSAIDs] like ibuprofen, and corticosteroids) used to treat chronic disease conditions knock out all the eicosanoids, it's commonly assumed that all eicosanoids are bad. Yet the good eicosanoids derived from DGLA are just as powerful as the bad eicosanoids.*

To understand how important the good eicosanoids are at the molecular level, let's take a closer look at one of the best known of the good eicosanoids that comes from DGLA—prostaglandin E_1, or PGE_1—and what it does in the body. First of all, PGE_1 performs a number of crucial jobs for the cardiovascular system. It inhibits the clumping of platelets, thus reducing the risk of blood clots. It helps blood vessels dilate, ensuring adequate blood flow to and from the heart and helping to combat the clogging effects of atherosclerosis. (Interestingly, that increased blood flow is why injections of PGE_1 are one of the primary treatments for impotence in men.) And it also helps cut down the body's manufacture of cholesterol in the liver.

PGE_1 has powerful effects on the immune system as well. It controls the release of *lymphokines*, the natural substances that "prime" the immune system to take action. It reduces the proliferation of immune-system cells, which can sometimes overreact and begin attacking other cells in the body. (This is essentially what happens in *autoimmune* diseases like rheumatoid arthritis.) It cuts down the release of histamine, thus helping to put the brakes on a wide variety of allergic reactions; and it reduces pain. PGE_1 also acts to combat inflammation.

In the endocrine system, PGE_1 stimulates the manufacture and

---

*There is one good eicosanoid that is derived from arachidonic acid: PGI_2, also known as prostacyclin. It's found primarily in the *endothelial* cells that line the inner walls of blood vessels. Unfortunately, there are no dietary means to increase prostacyclin levels without increasing the levels of bad eicosanoids.

secretion of vital hormones in the thyroid, adrenal, and pituitary glands—including human growth hormone. It controls the neurotransmitters, which act as the nervous system's chemical messengers. By increasing the uptake and release of these messengers, PGE_1 can reduce the need for sleep, and it can help alleviate depression. PGE_1 also acts as a powerful suppressor of insulin release from the pancreas—thereby setting up a positive feedback loop to help keep you in the Zone.

In the stomach, PGE_1 inhibits the secretion of acids, which if left unchecked create ulcers. In the respiratory system, it has a relaxing effect on tissues in the bronchial tubes, helping to reduce the intensity of asthma attacks.

I think you'll agree that for one substance that's an amazingly long job description. Now consider that PGE_1 is only one of many good eicosanoids, and you'll get an idea as to how ubiquitous they are in the body, and how absolutely crucial they are in keeping all of the body's machinery running smoothly.

STACKING THE DECK

Now let's put all this together. To reach the Zone and reap its health and performance rewards, you want to stack the eicosanoid deck in your favor. You want to ensure that your cells produce more good eicosanoids than bad ones. How do you do that? By tilting the balance of DGLA to arachidonic acid in your favor.

As I said earlier, the most consistent way to achieve this goal is to maintain the appropriate balance between your constant hormonal companions, insulin and glucagon. Too much insulin increases the activity of the delta 5 desaturase enzyme, the trigger for the increased production of arachidonic acid and bad eicosanoids.

Glucagon, on the other hand, decreases the activity of the delta 5 desaturase enzyme. This means that more and more DGLA piles up in the cell membranes, while at the same time the production of arachidonic acid goes down.

Think of all this as a sort of biological lottery. DGLA and arachidonic acid are the tickets, and they're being called in every minute. The more DGLA tickets and the fewer arachidonic acid tickets you have in each cell, the more likely you are to win the grand prize: the favorable balance of eicosanoids that spells optimal health and maximum performance.

But keep in mind: even when you win the eicosanoid lottery, you spend all your "winnings" in four to six hours. Four to six hours later, another lottery takes place—your next meal. I've said it before, but it's worth saying again: you're only hormonally as good as your last meal, and you're only as hormonally good as your next meal.

Controlling the macronutrient content of those meals is up to you—if you want to live in the Zone.

CHAPTER THIRTEEN

THE ZONE AND YOUR HEART

For the past forty years, Americans have been engaged in a life-and-death struggle with heart disease. Science and technology have provided us with an arsenal of powerful new weapons to fight this battle: drugs to lower blood pressure and cholesterol, coronary bypass surgery and heart transplants, pacemakers, and angioplasty, using both balloons and laser beams.

As a nation, we seem to exercise as never before—jogging, playing golf and tennis, lifting weights, and doing aerobics in every conceivable variety. And many of us, convinced by the media and the nutrition gurus, are eating diets that are supposed to be "heart-healthy."

If you read the newspapers or watch television, you're led to believe that all these measures are working. It seems that nearly every day the media trumpets the results of statistical studies showing that heart disease is on the decline, and that we're winning the war.

Yet, despite all this progress, the tragic truth is that heart disease remains by far the number-one killer of adults in this country. (In 1989, for example, heart disease killed more than 750,000 people, 50 percent more than the number-two leading cause of death, cancer.) In my own family, the numbers are far worse. My guess is that heart disease has also killed someone in your family, or someone close to you.

So we're really not making much progress in the war against heart disease. How can I say that? First, while the rates of death from cardiovascular disease have decreased, the number of heart attacks hasn't changed dramatically. In other words, Americans appear to be having the same number of heart attacks, it's just that the heart attacks aren't killing them as frequently.

Second, there's an alarming possibility that cardiovascular deaths have been systematically underreported. A recent study at Yale University indicated that there's been a difference in the reported cause of death and cause of death determined by autopsy. When the deaths were corrected to be in concert with autopsy results, the death rate from coronary disease in this sample didn't show the dramatic reduction that we hear so much about.

Finally, there's the growing epidemic of obesity in this country. No medical authority believes that increasing excess body fat is going to decrease the likelihood of a heart attack, yet that's exactly what's going on all over America—and it's happening at an accelerating rate. The simple truth is that the fatter you are the more likely you are to have a heart attack.

So if we're really not making that much progress in conquering heart disease, the next question, obviously, is why not? Here's a large part of the answer: *the way we're told to eat may be extremely hazardous to a healthy heart.* This is especially true of diets advocated by everyone from the Surgeon General of the United States to our local cable TV nutritionists—diets that emphasize eating small quantities of fat and protein and large amounts of carbohydrates, especially pasta. Many of us have tried or are still trying to adhere to these diets, reassured by the experts that eating this way will keep our arteries clear—if not actually reverse arterial disease—and keep our hearts pumping at uninterrupted full strength.

Sorry, but I have alarming news: *low-fat, high-carbohydrate diets are likely to promote heart disease—especially if you're genetically predisposed to a high insulin response to carbohydrates. If you're eating this way, you're putting yourself in danger—you're not minimizing your risk of heart disease, you're actually increasing that risk.*

RISK FACTORS FOR HEART DISEASE

All efforts to deal with heart disease in this country are based on the diagnosis and treatment of risk factors, which are associated with an increased likelihood of a heart attack. Many of these risk factors—obesity, high blood pressure, and high cholesterol, for example—are well known, and I'll get to them in a moment. For now, though, I'd like to talk about a risk factor that you've probably never heard of in the popular press. When I'm through, you'll understand why all those trendy high-carbohydrate diets may be increasing your risk of developing heart disease.

HYPERINSULINEMIA

What is that risk factor? *Hyperinsulinemia*. In fact, for the past twenty years, scientific evidence has been accumulating to suggest that *hyperinsulinemia is the risk factor that best predicts the likelihood of an eventual heart attack.*

For example: as I mentioned earlier, a 1987 study by a team of researchers at Stanford University showed that as many as 25 percent of an otherwise normal, healthy population—that's about 60 million Americans—respond genetically to excess dietary carbohydrate by producing too much insulin. I think it's highly possible that this subset of the U.S. population may make up nearly 100 percent of our heart-disease patients.

Look at the numbers: 25 percent of adult Americans—some sixty million people—have risk factors (such as high blood pressure and high cholesterol) associated with heart disease. This may well be the same sixty million people who have a genetic predisposition to an elevated insulin response to carbohydrates.

What's the connection between heart disease, the standard risk factors, and hyperinsulinemia? The answer is the overproduction of bad eicosanoids. Remember that insulin increases the production of bad eicosanoids, so the higher your blood insulin levels, the more bad eicosanoids your body produces.

Let's explore this in a little more detail. As we've seen, too much carbohydrate (and too little fat and protein to control the rate of entry of carbohydrates into the bloodstream) means an overproduction of insulin. Higher insulin levels enhance the activity of the enzyme (delta 5 desaturase) that converts DGLA (the building block for good eicosanoids) to arachidonic acid (the building block for bad eicosanoids). *This disturbance in normal eicosanoid balance is the primary molecular cause of heart disease.*

So here's the equation you should memorize if you're concerned about heart attacks: High-carbohydrate diet (especially if you are genetically predisposed to an elevated insulin response to carbohydrates) = more delta 5 desaturase activity = more arachidonic acid production = more bad eicosanoids = increased incidence of heart attacks.

To help you recall this equation, remember the rabbit story. You can inject virtually every one of the essential fatty acids (except arachidonic acid) into rabbits and nothing happens. (You can even inject the rabbits with cholesterol, and still nothing happens.) But if you inject the same amount of arachidonic acid into the rabbits, you'll get a scene right out of *The Andromeda Strain*. The arachidonic acid builds up in the rabbits' bloodstream, their blood clots almost instantaneously, and within three minutes they're dead.

But you don't have to inject arachidonic acid into the bloodstream to increase its levels. There's a slower, more relentless and insidious way: just keep eating a high-carbohydrate diet, and the resulting hyperinsulinemia may do it for you.

How can you tell if you're hyperinsulinemic? Take off all your clothes and look in the mirror. If you're fat and you're shaped like an apple, you're hyperinsulinemic, and you don't need a medical test to tell you. (It's also quite possible to be lean and have elevated insulin levels.) If you're hyperinsulinemic, you're producing too many bad eicosanoids and placing your heart in danger.

How do you deal with this? One way is to take aspirin for the rest of your life. That will reduce the production of bad eicosanoids. But bear in mind that taking aspirin itself is not a magic bullet. Aspirin also decreases the production of good eicosanoids, the hormonal key to cardiovascular health. A far better—and far more sophisticated way—to deal with hyperinsulinemia is to follow a Zone-favorable diet. Staying in the Zone will decrease your body's production of bad eicosanoids, and simultaneously increase its production of good ones. So remember: the balance of eicosanoids is the primary factor determining whether or not the heart stays healthy.

HIGH BLOOD PRESSURE

Hyperinsulinemia may be the greatest (and the least-known) risk factor for heart disease, but it's certainly not the only one. Millions of Americans also suffer from high blood pressure (hypertension), which promotes heart disease by damaging blood vessels or enlarging the heart itself.

There's another way to define hypertension. Like so many other disease states, it occurs when the body makes more bad eicosanoids than good ones. These bad eicosanoids cause the blood vessels to narrow. (Doctors call this *vasoconstriction*.) Good eicosanoids increase the diameter of blood vessels (*vasodilation*).

When blood vessels constrict—especially if the vessels are already narrowed by atherosclerosis—blood flow to the heart is compromised. This means angina, chest pains, and a vastly increased risk of eventual heart attack.

What narrows the arteries? Often it's a bad eicosanoid known as thromboxane A_2, which is an extremely powerful vasoconstricting agent. So the development of hypertension is really an indication of an inexorable buildup of thromboxane A_2.

Thromboxane A_2 is difficult, if not impossible, to measure. But it's easy to measure hypertension. It's determined by your blood pressure, which consists of two numbers. The higher number is called the systolic blood pressure, the lower is called the diastolic blood pressure. The diastolic number measures the pressure when the heart is not forcing blood through the cardiovascular system.

The systolic number can best be thought of as an indicator of the elasticity of the blood vessels, while the diastolic number indicates whether or not the vessels are partially clogged. If they are partially clogged, it's like bad plumbing, making it much more difficult for blood to flow through the vessels, hence more likely to clot.

Of the two numbers, the diastolic is usually of greater concern to a physician. It can reveal hypertension in varying degrees of severity. A diastolic reading of 105 (the lower number of your blood pressure reading) is considered moderate hypertension, indicating that some type of cardiovascular damage is likely to occur eventually if the hypertension is left untreated. If the diastolic reading reaches 115, the hypertension is considered severe. Serious damage, such as a stroke, is imminent. A diastolic reading of 130 is called malignant hypertension. This is extremely dangerous and immediately life-threatening.

There's no question that when diastolic blood pressures are in the 105 to 130 range, immediate treatment with antihypertensive drugs is imperative. But the number of patients with these severely elevated diastolic readings represents only a small portion of the defined hypertensive population. The population with only moderate hypertension—a diastolic blood pressure between 90 and 105—accounts for the vast bulk of antihypertensive drug sales.

There's no doubt that clinical studies have conclusively shown that for people with more extreme levels of hypertension (greater than 105), drug intervention is life saving. But what are the effects of drug intervention on the vast majority of patients taking hypertensive drugs—the patients with moderate hypertension?

This question led to one of the largest clinical trials ever sponsored by the U.S. government: the Multiple Risk Factor Intervention Trial, or MR. FIT. The MR. FIT study was a ten-year, $115 million trial started in 1973. More than 12,000 high-risk males were split into two groups. Those in the control group, called the Usual Care Group, were simply told they were at risk for heart disease, and that they should try to take care of themselves. Members of the other group, the Special Intervention Group, were given antihypertensive medication (diuretics) in an attempt to reduce their blood pressure. They were also provided with aggressive diet counseling.

This part of the study looked like a great success: 87 percent of the Special Intervention Group were able to reduce diastolic pressure to below 105, and 66 percent were able to get diastolic blood pressure into the normal range (less than 90).

But the only number that really counts is the reduction in death rates. Well, ten years later, when the study looked at death rates, they found no difference between the two groups.

Another large-scale study in Britain in 1985 confirmed this unsettling conclusion. This time the numbers were even larger (more than 17,000), and included both men and women with diastolic blood pressure between 90 and 105. In this five-year trial, while there was a decrease in the number of strokes, there wasn't any difference in the number of heart attacks or the number of deaths between the two groups. In other words, even though blood pressure was reduced, the overall mortality hadn't changed. In fact—and this is a very disturbing trend—the women in the group who were treated with drugs and diet counseling appeared to be dying at a greater rate than women in the control group who got no treatment at all.

It has only recently been understood that while the antihypertensive drugs used in these studies—drugs that are still widely used today—do cause significant reductions in blood pressure, they also cause an increase in insulin levels. I suspect that the lack of effect on overall mortality in the drug-treatment group may be due to an increase in bad eicosanoid production caused by increased insulin levels.

Even though blood pressure was being controlled, I suspect that increasing bad eicosanoid production—especially of thromboxane A_2—increased the likelihood of platelet aggregation and blood clotting. The end result: the negative effect of bad eicosanoids on the overall progression of heart disease had overwhelmed the positive effect of reducing hypertension.

Remember—my definition of disease is simply the body making more bad eicosanoids and less good ones. So, if bad eicosanoids, such as thromboxane A_2, can promote hypertension, is there any evidence that good eicosanoids can reduce it?

The answer is yes. One of the best-known and most-studied of the good eicosanoids is prostaglandin E_1 (PGE_1). PGE_1 and other good eicosanoids help put the clamps on the secretion of insulin, and that in turn helps limit the production of bad eicosanoids. Besides reducing insulin levels, good eicosanoids also promote vasodilation, so that instead of narrowing, blood vessels actually widen. The combined result: blood pressure goes down, and so does the risk of heart disease.

Do you need drugs to increase the production of good eicosanoids like PGE_1? No. Simply limit the production of bad eicosanoids (like thromboxane A_2) while simultaneously increasing the production of good eicosanoids like PGE_1, and you'll automatically bring your blood pressure down. To accomplish that, all you need is a Zone-favorable diet.

CHOLESTEROL

Reduce your cholesterol and be free of heart trouble. That's been the battle cry for the war on heart disease. But the rules for the war on cholesterol are constantly changing. When the war first started about fifteen years ago, the villain was total cholesterol. Then the experts focused on "bad" cholesterol—LDL and VLDL. These days, it's the ratio of total cholesterol to "good," or HDL cholesterol.

But the one question that no one seems to have asked is "If cholesterol is such a villain, why does the body make so much of it?" The truth is that cholesterol is essential to life. It's the primary structural component of every cell in the body. Remove even 30 percent or less of the cholesterol in a red blood cell, and its membrane disintegrates.

Cholesterol is also the building block for every steroid hormone known to man. Cortisol, adrenaline, testosterone, estrogen, dehydro-epiandrone (DHEA), etc.—they're all made from cholesterol. Without cholesterol, a great many of your hormonal control systems would immediately grind to a halt.

The bottom line is that you need cholesterol to survive. Decreasing its levels too much may have devastating consequences.

Of course, the strong consensus of the medical community is that too much cholesterol has the same effect: it increases overall mortality. So reducing cholesterol in those who have too much of it should decrease mortality. Does it? Sadly, the answer is no. There's no association between high cholesterol and death from heart disease in people over seventy, the group in which a lifetime of high cholesterol should theoretically do the most damage.

Let's look at the facts, beginning with studies that have used drugs to lower cholesterol. One of the first of these trials, conducted in the early 1970s, used the drug clofibrate to lower cholesterol. Yet even though cholesterol levels were reduced, the number of deaths in the people treated with clofibrate was actually 29 percent greater than in the control group in which people took only a placebo.

In 1987 came the famous Helsinki Heart Study, in which a different cholesterol-lowering drug, gemfibrozil, was given to more than four thousand patients. The good news was that the drug did lower cholesterol by as much as 10 percent, and the number of heart attacks was reduced by 35 percent. (In fact, the medical community used those numbers to demonstrate the critical need to lower everyone's cholesterol.) Unfortunately, the treatment group had more total deaths than the control group, which got only the placebo. Overall mortality had not changed at all.

Still, the Helsinki study apparently whetted the medical community's appetite for more aggressive use of new cholesterol-lowering drugs—at least in people with very high cholesterol levels. Among the first of these drugs was lovastatin, which acts on the enzyme that regulates cholesterol production in the liver (more about this enzyme in a moment). Lovastatin, it turns out, has an even greater cholesterol-lowering capability than gemfibrozil. As a result, it's been so aggressively marketed that it's now among the biggest-selling drugs in the world.

But hold on: lovastatin has been shown by a number of investigators to have a very disturbing side effect—it increases the patients' levels of arachidonic acid. You'll recall that arachidonic acid is the same fatty acid that's the building block for bad eicosanoids like thromboxane A_2.

However, newer versions of these cholesterol-lowering drugs, such as simvastatin and pravastatin, have shown early promise in both lowering cholesterol and reducing overall mortality. In 1994 a five-year trial with over 4,000 patients using simvastatin did produce heartening results in both respects. However, there's an important caveat: this study excluded patients with high triglycerides, which are an indication of hyperinsulinemia—the primary risk factor for predicting heart attacks. But this critique was eliminated with another study using pravastatin. This large-scale study (6,000 patients over five years) showed a 33 percent reduction in overall cardiovascular mortality in patients with no previous existing heart disease, and a 22 percent reduction in overall mortality. However, the reduction in overall mortality was just barely significant.

While the newest cholesterol-lowering drugs reduce overall mortality from heart disease, what about cholesterol-lowering diets? Over a twenty-year period only one of six studies—the Oslo study— showed any decrease in cardiovascular mortality with a cholesterol-lowering diet (and this study included an aggressive antismoking component). But even this study showed no decrease in overall mortality. Another factor: in the Oslo study, the average cholesterol level of the patients was well over 300 mg/dl, an incredibly high level demanding immediate medical attention.

But patients with cholesterol levels greater than 300 mg constitute only a small percentage of the high-cholesterol population. The vast majority of these patients considered high-risk have much lower cholesterol levels, between 240 and 300 mg/dl. *No diet study has ever been conducted to demonstrate a decrease in mortality in these patients.*

Even so, many experts will tell you that the way to lower cholesterol is simply to avoid it in your diet. Unfortunately, the amount of cholesterol you eat has a relatively low impact on the amount of cholesterol in your bloodstream. The truth is that more than 80 percent of your daily cholesterol production comes not from diet but from your own liver.

The enzyme that controls cholesterol synthesis in the liver is called *HMG CoA reductase.* (In fact, the 1985 Nobel Prize in Medicine was awarded for understanding how this one enzyme controls the rate at which the liver produces cholesterol.) This the same enzyme that these new cholesterol-lowering drugs (lovastatin, simvastin, and pravastatin) all inhibit, and that is why they lower cholesterol levels. By now it shouldn't be surprising that, like all key enzymes, HMG CoA reductase is under hormonal control—in particular, under the control of insulin and glucagon. Insulin activates HMG CoA reductase, causing the liver to make more cholesterol. Glucagon inhibits the enzyme, so that the liver makes less cholesterol.

What else inhibits the activity of HMG CoA reductase? Good eicosanoids. Sound familiar?

So let's say you're eating one of these trendy, recommended diets that are low in cholesterol and high in carbohydrates. If you're genetically predisposed to have an elevated insulin response to carbohydrates, then you're doing everything in your power to increase the body's production of cholesterol—even though there's almost no cholesterol in your diet.

No wonder that dietary intervention to reduce cholesterol rarely seems to work. That's because no diet other than a Zone-favorable diet addresses what's really controlling your cholesterol levels: eicosanoids.

Here's one example. A cardiovascular patient came to me after being on a radically high-carbohydrate diet. The diet affected this patient in exactly the wrong way. His levels of triglycerides and cholesterol rose to highly elevated levels (650 mg/dl and 229 mg/dl respectively), and his good HDL cholesterol level dropped (to 34 mg/dl). These were sure indications that the patient was developing insulin resistance.

After discussing the situation with me, he changed to a Zone-favorable diet. At the same time, his doctor put him on simvastatin—

the same drug that had gotten the recent good press. Within six months his lipid profile had improved dramatically. His triglycerides dropped from 650 to 108, his total cholesterol dropped from 229 to 152, and his HDL cholesterol increased from 34 to 49.

Was it the diet or was it the drug? The patient stopped taking the simvastatin, but continued on the Zone-favorable diet. While his total cholesterol did rise slightly, to 175, his triglycerides continued to drop to 101 and his HDL cholesterol further increased to 52. This patient's story is a dramatic indication that cholesterol levels are ultimately determined by eicosanoid balance, which is controlled by the food you eat.

OBESITY AND TYPE II DIABETES

If the pharmaceutical war on hypertension and high cholesterol has not improved overall mortality, it did reduce blood pressure and cholesterol. But the battle against the fourth major risk factor—obesity and its all-too-frequent outcome, Type II diabetes—has been a totally lost cause. Not only are Americans in general getting fatter, but so are cardiovascular patients.

If you're overweight, you should be concerned not just about your excess fat but also about the *location* of that fat. If you have abdominal obesity (you look like an apple), as opposed to being fat in general (you look like a pear), your risk for a heart attack is dramatically increased. Why? As we said earlier, abdominal obesity is a dead giveaway: you almost certainly have elevated levels of insulin. And remember, hyperinsulinemia is the primary risk factor for heart attacks.

Hyperinsulinemia is also the clinical definition of Type II diabetes. This form of the disease, also known as adult-onset diabetes, because it generally appears after age forty, accounts for more than 90 percent of the diabetic population. Unfortunately, Type II diabetic patients are among those at the highest risk for heart attack because of their elevated insulin levels. Keep in mind that elevated insulin is why people get fat in the first place. (To make matters worse, elevated insulin levels also cause the body to increase the production of arachidonic acid, a cardiovascular patient's worst nightmare.)

Ironically, even though their levels of insulin are already too high, Type II patients are usually treated with drugs that further increase their insulin levels. (If that doesn't work, they're eventually given injections of insulin, which has the same result.) Wait a minute: why *increase* their insulin levels? Because they have a condition known as insulin resistance.

In this condition, cells become less receptive to insulin. More and more circulating insulin is needed to reduce blood-sugar levels. This is a case of winning the battle (reducing blood sugar), but losing the war (increasing insulin levels).

Obviously, insulin resistance greatly increases the potential for developing Type II diabetes. How do you recognize that potential? You're fat with an apple shape (indicating high insulin levels), have high blood levels of triglycerides, low blood levels of HDL, and hypertension. (This deadly quartet is also known as Syndrome X, and was first elucidated by George Reaven at Stanford University in the mid 1980s.) Since America is getting fatter and older (remember, the incidence of Type II diabetes increases with age), it is estimated by the year 2000 there will be twenty-five million Type II diabetics in this country.

The best way to treat Type II diabetes and the hyperinsulinemia that causes it is to target that excess body fat. If the accumulation of excess body fat is caused by hyperinsulinemia, then reduction of excess body fat should decrease insulin resistance and reduce circulating insulin levels. When insulin levels are reduced, arachidonic acid levels should also decline. If you reduce arachidonic acid levels, the overproduction of bad eicosanoids, such as thromboxane A_2, should be reduced. And if the overproduction of bad eicosanoids is reduced, then the likelihood of having a heart attack is greatly reduced.

This train of molecular events explains why losing body fat has such a dramatic impact on reducing blood pressure, high cholesterol levels, and Type II diabetes. Every cardiologist knows that when patients lose excess body fat, it's as if the hand of God touched them. If their patients lose excess body fat, then the primary risk factors for heart disease will disappear virtually overnight.

Why? Because when you boil it all down, the development of each of these risk factors is a consequence of being out of the Zone for extended periods of time. Put it another way: losing excess body fat—

the best way to reduce risk factors associated with heart disease—only occurs if you're in the Zone.

Yet one of the greatest failures of twentieth-century cardiovascular medicine is its inability to find a way to reduce excess body fat and keep it off. Diet should be the desired method, but diets have continually failed. Why have they failed? *Because the recommended dietary programs for cardiovascular patients and for people trying to lose excess body fat in general are in constant violation of the rules needed to reach the Zone.*

The only way to achieve the goal of permanent fat loss is to live as much of your life as possible in the Zone. If you can do that, you have done the most important thing in your power to reduce your risk of dying from heart disease.

How do you get that lifelong passport to the Zone? You already know the answer: through the food you eat.

SMOKING AND DRINKING

Smoking and drinking are among the best-known behavioral risk factors that impact heart disease. Let's look at smoking first. During the time a person smokes, he or she incurs a tremendous increased risk of a heart attack. But if the person quits smoking, within a few years the risk will be greatly diminished.

The act of smoking generates a tremendous increase of free radicals. You'll remember that free radicals deplete the body's natural reserves of antioxidants, and this in turn exposes the essential fatty acids that are the building blocks of eicosanoids to free-radical destruction. Once a person stops smoking, the increased exposure to excess free radicals stops. Since the body is constantly renewing itself, after a few years the impact of prior smoking on the future likelihood of having a heart attack is minimal.

There's also recent research indicating that smoking is associated with an increase in insulin resistance. That means a corresponding increase in hyperinsulinemia, the primary risk factor for predicting the likelihood of a heart attack. It may be that once you stop smoking the amount of insulin in your bloodstream declines to more healthful levels.

What about alcohol? In moderation, it's good for you. Take the

French paradox. Nutritionists hate the French because they have low rates of heart disease, but they still manage to have a good time. They eat a high-fat diet, they don't exercise, and they drink wine.

One of those factors must explain their low rates of heart disease. It turns out it's probably the wine. In moderate amounts, alcohol increases the production of good eicosanoids. This increase in good eicosanoids brings a subsequent decrease in platelet aggregation.

You have to be careful, though. In higher amounts alcohol increases the production of bad eicosanoids. So how much alcohol is moderate? About one glass of wine (especially red wine) per day. This is not to say that if you don't drink at all you ought to take it up. But if you drink, do so in moderation.

To sum up: both these environmental risk factors for heart disease are under your control. One, smoking, is very dangerous and should be avoided at all costs. The other, alcohol, is potentially good, but only in moderation.

ARTERIAL BLOCKAGE: BLOOD CLOTS AND ATHEROSCLEROSIS

Up to now I've been talking about factors that increase your risk for heart disease and life-threatening heart attacks. But in most cases, the actual trigger (or *proximal cause*, to use the medical term) of heart attack is the failure of blood flow to the heart due to a blocked artery.

Blood carries oxygen to the heart. If the heart doesn't get enough oxygen, the heart muscle cells die. Heart muscle cells are like any muscle cell: the ones you're born with are the only ones you get. If the heart muscles die because of a lack of oxygen, they won't be replaced.

There are a number of factors that can lead to the arterial blockage that ultimately kills the heart by cutting off its oxygen supply. These factors often work in combination, but for the moment let's take them one at a time.

Platelet aggregation is the clumping together of circulating platelets in the bloodstream to form clots. Under some circumstances, platelet aggregation is a good thing. If you're cut, for example, you want your blood to form clots to prevent you from bleeding to death.

But what happens if platelets begin to clump at the wrong time? If the platelet clot is large enough, it can clog the artery entirely, especially if the artery is already narrowed by atherosclerosis. (More about atherosclerosis in a moment.) When the artery is blocked entirely, that chokes off blood (and therefore oxygen supply) to the heart, and brings on a life-threatening heart attack.

What causes platelets to aggregate at the wrong time? Bad eicosanoids, especially thromboxane A_2. In fact, thromboxane A_2 is the most powerful blood-clotting agent known. Remember too that thromboxane A_2 causes the blood vessels to narrow (vasoconstriction). Not only that, but bad eicosanoids like thromboxane A_2 stimulate the multiplication of abnormal smooth muscle cells that make up a layer of the artery wall. When these cells multiply too much, they cause the development of the atherosclerotic lesions that narrow the blood vessels.

Put these three effects—blood clotting, abnormal smooth muscle cell proliferation, and vasoconstriction—together, and you have a powerful triple whammy that can easily bring on a heart attack.

If bad eicosanoids can promote life-threatening arterial blockage, can good eicosanoids keep that blockage from forming, or help bypass it if it does form? The answer to both these questions may well be yes. First of all, good eicosanoids like PGE_1 are powerful vasodilators. They inhibit the platelet aggregation that leads to blood clots, and they slow the proliferation of smooth muscle cells that can contribute to atherosclerosis.

In fact, a team of scientists in Kassel, Germany, showed just how powerful good eicosanoids can be in this regard. The German researchers were treating a diabetic patient who had gangrene in one leg, caused by a severe blockage in one of her arteries. The usual treatment in such cases is amputation.

But instead of undertaking the standard amputation, the German team gave the patient an injection of PGE_1. This, they thought, might increase the diameter of the clogged artery enough so that blood could flow past the blockage, renewing the supply of oxygen to her leg muscles.

The result? Within one hour after the injection of PGE_1, there was an increase in blood flow. An angiogram 12 days later showed a dramatic (nearly 500 percent) increase in the diameter of the artery.

Oxygen transfer was increased, and the leg was saved.

Even though they can be caused by a long-term buildup of bad eicosanoids, the blood clots that threaten life and limb tend to come on suddenly. More insidious—and, in some ways, more difficult to treat—is *atherosclerosis:* the narrowing and hardening of the arteries caused by a buildup of fatty deposits known as plaques. These plaques are dangerous not only because they constrict the arteries, but because pieces of them can break off and travel to the heart itself, causing a heart attack.

Now, an artery can be up to 75 percent blocked by atherosclerotic lesions and still provide normal blood flow so that you can do your daily tasks. Still, the likelihood of a platelet clot cutting off the flow is higher than normal because of the smaller size of the blocked artery. So if you can reverse the atherosclerotic buildup in the blocked artery, you should decrease the likelihood that a small clot will block the artery and cause a heart attack. (Of course, if you make a big clot, then it really doesn't matter how much you have regressed the lesion, the artery will still be blocked.)

It's obviously worthwhile to try to reverse atherosclerosis. In fact, this reversal has been the Holy Grail of the quest to conquer heart disease. Theoretically, there are two ways to accomplish reversal of atherosclerosis: drugs and diet.

A good example of the first approach was the Cholesterol Lowering Atherosclerotic Study (CLAS), which was published in 1987. Since cholesterol is one of the major components of the plaques that cause atherosclerosis, the idea was to try to achieve regression using a combination of cholesterol-lowering drugs—in this case colestipol and high doses of niacin.

There were more than 180 patients in the CLAS study. Half the patients were given an aggressive schedule of the two cholesterol-lowering drugs. After two years, the drugs had had no effect on the atherosclerotic lesions in most of the patients (84 percent). But there was some degree of regression in 16 percent of the patients.

Obviously, a 16 percent success rate sounds a lot better than saying you've had an 84 percent rate of failure. Nonetheless, even this very limited success in regression would represent a major advance if overall mortality were decreased. That's the real question: Is the change significant enough to help prevent heart attacks and reduce mortality? Unfortunately, the CLAS study didn't address this question, so at this time no one knows.

In 1994, researchers published a study in which a combination of diet and the newest cholesterol-lowering drug (simvastatin) were used to try to achieve regression of atherosclerotic lesions. Although the patients treated this way did show a small decrease in blockage (about 2.5 percent), there was no change in clinical outcome after four years of treatment. This lack of clinical benefit in spite of lesion regression was also observed in two earlier studies—the MARS and CCAIT studies—using drugs similar to simvastatin.

What is known, however, is that the patients who got the drugs had significantly more adverse medical side effects than the patients who got only a placebo. Both groups had equal numbers of adverse cardiovascular events. Actually, this isn't surprising. Drugs are known to cause side effects that could possibly eliminate any benefits resulting from regression of an atherosclerotic lesion.

The bottom line: drugs have their problems, especially if you have to take them for the rest of your life. And that includes the drug most widely used to combat heart disease—aspirin.

ASPIRIN

Aspirin doesn't lower cholesterol. It doesn't lower blood pressure. It doesn't lower high blood sugar in Type II diabetics. It doesn't reduce excess body fat. But it works.

As we've seen, there are remarkably few drug-intervention studies for standard hypertension and elevated cholesterol levels that have been shown to significantly reduce total mortality . But there's no question that in people with preexisting heart disease the number of heart attacks is significantly reduced by taking aspirin—and so is the overall death rate.

But does an otherwise healthy population get the same benefits from aspirin? This question was answered in the famous Physicians Heart Study in 1988. This landmark study was conducted with more than 22,000 physicians who had no evidence of heart disease. Half the physicians took 160 mg of aspirin (half a standard tablet) every day; the other half took a placebo. When the study was concluded, the researchers found that the incidence of heart attacks was 40 percent greater in the placebo group—a major difference.

Unfortunately, there were no differences in the total mortality rates after four years. Still, it may be that four years is simply too short a period of time to see long-term differences in overall mortality.

Or there could be another explanation. Remember that aspirin's only effect is on eicosanoids. On the one hand, it reduces the production of bad eicosanoids that promote platelet aggregation, such as thromboxane A_2. Unfortunately, at the same time aspirin also reduces the production of good eicosanoids, like PGE_1, that prevent platelet aggregation. This two-edged sword may well explain why the overall mortality rates of the Physicians Heart Study using a population with no initial sign of heart disease did not change during the four-year period of the study.

Although the jury is still out on the daily use of aspirin's effect on overall mortality in healthy people, the aspirin studies have given a unique insight into what should be the ideal intervention for heart disease. The ideal intervention for heart disease would simply consist of reducing the overproduction of bad eicosanoids, while simultaneously increasing the production of good eicosanoids.

You can do that with a Zone-favorable diet.

THE ZONE-FAVORABLE TYPE II DIABETIC STUDY

So far, I've made some strong statements about drug and diet trials and cardiovascular outcome. Remember: the only statistic that truly counts is mortality. Is the drug or the diet preventing early death or not? From that point of view, as we've seen, most intervention studies have come up short of their promise.

In the absence of mortality data, is there anything that indicates that a Zone-favorable diet would be beneficial for a cardiovascular patient? I believe the answer is yes. Throughout this book, my constant theme has been the importance of controlling insulin so as to maintain a favorable eicosanoid balance. So the question is: can a Zone-favorable diet significantly lower insulin levels in cardiovascular patients?

In 1994 I conducted a pilot study in collaboration with a respected cardiology group in the greater Boston area, a team that had considerable experience conducting clinical trials with major drug companies. All clinical studies should be compared to something. If your goal is to show how diet affects hyperinsulinemia, you should start with patients who are already hyperinsulinemic. The ideal patient group: Type II diabetics, who by definition are hyperinsulinemic.

We enrolled 15 Type II diabetic patients, and randomized them into two groups. One group followed a Zone-favorable diet, and the other group followed the dietary recommendations of the American Diabetes Association (ADA). The critical difference between these diets lies in their protein-to-carbohydrate ratios. A Zone-favorable diet has a protein-to-carbohydrate ratio of 0.75 (three grams of protein for every four grams of carbohydrate) while the ADA diet has a ratio of 0.33 (1 gram of protein for every three grams of carbohydrate).

Compliance—getting the patients to eat what you want them to eat—is the key to any dietary study. What better way to improve compliance than to package some of the meals as a candy bar? For this study I used a newer version of the experimental prototype "candy bar" I had used in my earlier weight-loss study, described in Chapter 2. You may recall that the prototype "candy bar" was actually a Zone-favorable meal in disguise. It contained two blocks of protein, two blocks of carbohydrate, two blocks of fat, and all the micronutrients needed for eicosanoid formation.

After eight weeks, both groups were analyzed for changes in their diabetic status. There are a number of factors that determine this status, but the most important for the physician is the patients' long-term blood-sugar control. This is measured by the amount of a substance called *glycosylated hemoglobin* found in the red blood cells.

The higher the levels of glycosylated hemoglobin, the higher the risk for cardiovascular complications. If blood-sugar levels are consistently elevated, the glycosylated hemoglobin reacts with proteins to create substances known as AGEs (AGE stands for *advanced glycosylated endproducts*). These AGEs are "sticky," and adhere to arterial vessels in the heart, the microvessels in the hands and feet, and the vessels in the eye. In doing so, they contribute to the buildup of plaques that can cause atherosclerosis and promote heart attacks.

Another important factor in determining diabetic status is fasting insulin levels (that is, insulin levels measured after allowing for any food in the system to be digested and absorbed). The higher these levels, the greater the extent of hyperinsulinemia. Since elevated insulin levels encourage the production of bad eicosanoids, and bad eicosanoids stimulate even more insulin secretion, this sets up a very unpleasant, not to say dangerous, feedback loop for the patient.

So my study was designed to test the effect of a Zone-favorable diet on these critical determinants of Type II diabetes. The results are shown in Table 13-1, and graphically in Figure 13-1. After eight weeks there were already statistically significant differences in the two groups. The patients on a Zone-favorable diet had large reductions in glycosylated hemoglobin, and, even more important, in fasting insulin.

When insulin drops, that usually causes two other heart-healthy

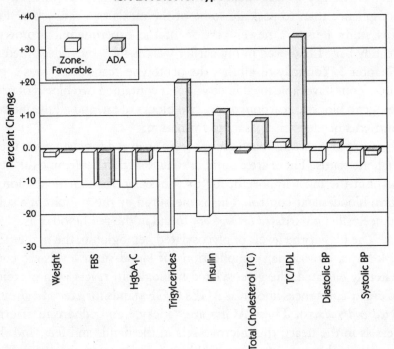

8-Week Results of a Zone-Favorable Diet vs. ADA Diet for Type II Diabetics

Figure 13-1

events: a drop in triglycerides and a drop in blood pressure (especially diastolic blood pressure). This is exactly what happened in the Zone-favorable group.

These patients got still another cardiovascular benefit: they lost weight. In fact, they averaged about one pound of weight loss per week—exactly the amount of weight loss recommended as sensible by the American Diabetes Association. Even better, all the weight loss on the Zone-favorable diet was pure excess body fat.

The patients were definitely in the Zone.

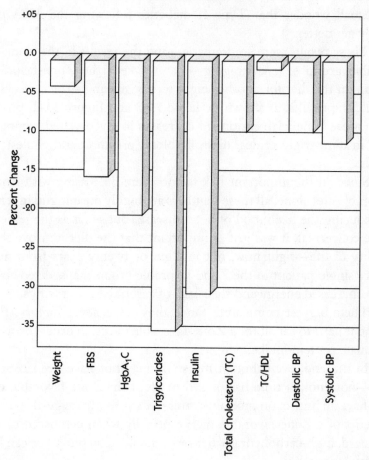

16-Week Results of a Zone-Favorable Diet for Type II Diabetics

Figure 13-2

In the group that followed the American Diabetes Association (ADA) diet, the results were not as favorable. In this group, insulin levels actually rose, with a corresponding increase in the levels of triglycerides. That's exactly what happened to patients following a high-carbohydrate, low-fat diet. It should be noted that the reduction of the fasting glucose levels of the patients following the ADA diet was achieved only with a compensatory increase in fasting insulin levels. This extremely adverse consequence is confirmed by the rising triglyceride levels, which are usually indicative of insulin resistance. There was also a dramatic increase in the ratio of total cholesterol to HDL cholesterol. Equally bad, the patients on the ADA diet experienced no weight loss.

Small wonder that Type II diabetics following the ADA diet rarely get better.

These results were so dramatic—and the results in the Zone-favorable group so encouraging—that we kept the Zone-favorable group on the diet for another eight weeks, making sixteen weeks in total. The results, as shown in Table 13-2 and Figure 13-2, proved even more beneficial: continued decreases in glycosylated hemoglobin, insulin, triglycerides, diastolic blood pressure, and cholesterol levels.

Since all the important risk factors were decreasing with Zone-favorable diet alone, all these numbers are highly meaningful in terms of reducing the likelihood of heart disease. But as far as the patients were concerned, it was just as important that the diet improve their quality of life—right now, not just ten or twenty years from now. Every single patient in the Zone-favorable group rhapsodized about their increased energy and their lack of carbohydrate cravings.

Their biggest complaint? Since they were never hungry, they found it hard to eat all their Zone-favorable meals, in order to ensure adequate protein intake.

In the end, even though my study may not have been conclusive—not enough time has passed to see if the Zone-favorable diet will have an impact on mortality rates—it's strongly suggestive of the benefits of a Zone-favorable diet; especially when compared to the standard, high-carbohydrate diet recommended by the American Diabetes Association.

Other studies are now appearing that support what we found in

TABLE 13-1

8-Week Comparison of Defined Diets on Type II Diabetic Patients

Zone-Favorable Diet: n=8 (5 males, 3 females)
Age = 60 ± 2 years

PARAMETER	INITIAL	WEEK 8	CHANGE	% CHANGE*	STATISTICAL SIGNIFICANCE**
Total weight	224	217	−7	−3	$p < 0.025$
Total fat	80	72	−8	−9	$p < 0.01$
Fasting glucose	201	176	−25	−12	n.s.
HgbA$_1$C	9.2	7.9	−1.3	−14	$p < 0.05$
Triglycerides	253	184	−69	−27	$p < 0.05$
Fasting insulin	30	24	−6	−20	n.s.
Systolic BP	133	128	−5	−4	$p < 0.01$
Diastolic BP	82	77	−5	−6	n.s.
Total					
Cholesterol	220	218	−2	−1	n.s.
Total chol/HDL	5.8	6.0	+0.2	+3	n.s.

PARAMETER	INITIAL	WEEK 8	CHANGE	% CHANGE*	STATISTICAL SIGNIFICANCE**
American Diabetes Association Diet: n=7 (2 males, 5 females) Age = 63 ± 4 years					
Total weight	216	215	–1	0	n.s.
Total fat	79	78	–1	–1	n.s.
Fasting glucose	206	181	–25	–12	n.s.
HgbA$_1$C	9.0	8.6	–0.4	–4	p < 0.05
Triglycerides	217	260	+43	+20	n.s.
Fasting insulin	40	45	+5	+12	n.s.
Systolic BP	138	141	+3	+2	n.s.
Diastolic BP	79	77	–2	–2	n.s.
Total					
Cholesterol	217	234	+17	+8	p < 0.05
Total chol/HDL	5.2	6.9	+1.7	+33	p < 0.025

*compared to initial values

**paired t-test

TABLE 13-2

16-Week Effects of A Zone-Favorable Diet on Type II Diabetic Patients

Zone-Favorable Diet: n=8 (5 males, 3 females)
Age = 60 ± 2 years

PARAMETER	INITIAL	WEEK 16	CHANGE*	% CHANGE*	STATISTICAL SIGNIFICANCE**
Weight	224	216	-8	-4	p < 0.25
Total fat	80	73	-7	-9	p < 0.01
Fasting glucose	201	171	-30	-15	n.s.
HgbA$_1$C	9.2	7.4	-1.8	-20	p < 0.05
Triglycerides	253	165	-88	-35	p < 0.05
Insulin	30	21	-9	-30	n.s.
Systolic BP	133	121	-12	-9	p < 0.01
Diastolic BP	82	73	-9	-11	p < 0.025
Total cholesterol	220	200	-20	-9	n.s.
Total chol/HDL	5.8	5.7	-0.1	-2	n.s.

*compared to initial values

**paired t-test

our pilot study. One such trial, from the University of Naples, Italy, in 1992, showed that within fifteen days there were statistically significant reductions in blood insulin levels, triglycerides, and insulin resistance in patients on a Zone-favorable diet compared to the ADA diet. (Unlike our study, in which the patients were free-living individuals—and thus required to make their own meals—the Italian study took place in a metabolic ward, where each meal was rigorously controlled. By using the experimental candy bars to replace one meal and two snacks each day, we were able to get the type of patient compliance usually found only in a hospital ward study.)

Taken together, our pilot study and the Italian trial strongly indicate that a Zone-favorable diet can reduce insulin levels without reliance on drugs. Since high levels of insulin are the primary risk factor associated with heart disease, I hope that physicians will now reconsider the hormonal consequences of the high-carbohydrate diets they currently recommend to their patients.

RESTENOSIS

Every year, millions of Americans undergo angioplasty, a procedure in which clogged arteries are opened by tiny balloons, by whirring blades, or by laser beams. In as many as half of all angioplasty patients, cells in the artery walls soon start to multiply out of control, so that within weeks the arteries close up again.

This unfortunate process is known as *restenosis*. As if you hadn't guessed it by now, there's evidence that eicosanoids play a role in this event. An overproduction of bad eicosanoids appears to accelerate restenosis, making arteries reclog even faster and more thoroughly than before the angioplasty procedure. This leaves the patient in worse cardiovascular shape than ever. One more black mark for bad eicosanoids. If you are going to undergo angioplasty, I would recommend starting on a Zone-favorable diet before the operation and staying on it afterward.

THE ZONE, EICOSANOIDS, AND YOUR HEART

It's obvious that, taken as a whole, excessive amounts of bad eicosanoids are bad for the heart, while good eicosanoids can help keep the heart in great shape. So strategies that tip the balance in favor of good eicosanoids—and getting into the Zone—should be powerful tools in the war against heart disease.

If you're trying to prevent heart disease—or even if you already have it—there are a number of eicosanoid-modulating strategies you might consider. One is to take aspirin for the rest of your life. In proper doses, aspirin can knock out bad eicosanoids at a slightly faster rate than it knocks out good eicosanoids.

But taking aspirin is a tricky game to play, sort of like lighting a cigarette with a stick of dynamite. You can do it, but you must be very careful. No one yet knows what the "proper" dose of aspirin is, especially over a long period of time. And too much aspirin can suppress the production of *all* eicosanoids, good and bad.

So, since long-term aspirin use may be the biological equivalent of a loose cannon, why not take the safer way to control eicosanoid balance and thus reduce the risk of heart attack? Use the ultimate eicosanoid-controlling drug: food.

If you already have heart disease, the first thing you need to do is cut out all foods that provide arachidonic acid directly to the body, and thus lead to the increased production of bad eicosanoids such as thromboxane A_2. Three major culprits are organ meats (like liver), fatty cuts of red meat, and egg yolks—they're all rich in arachidonic acid. (If you want to be on the safe side, cut out all red meat.) One added tip for the cardiovascular patient: eat lots of salmon. It's rich in the activated omega-3 fatty acid (EPA) that provides another way to prevent any potential buildup of arachidonic acid.

Cutting out all arachidonic acid–rich foods will help reduce the production of heart-damaging bad eicosanoids. But to truly turn food into a wonder drug against heart disease, we want our diets to boost the production of good eicosanoids at the same time.

If you're not a cardiovascular patient, but want to prevent yourself from becoming one, follow the same rules. An ounce of prevention (following a Zone-favorable diet) is worth a pound of cure (the standard cardiovascular drugs or surgery you can otherwise expect). The bottom line: maintaining a favorable balance of eicosanoids will greatly reduce your risk of a heart attack. In other words, keeping your eicosanoids in balance can save your life.

CHAPTER FOURTEEN

CANCER AND THE ZONE

For the past twenty years, the medical establishment has been waging a highly publicized "War against Cancer." Yet most scientists engaged in that war will admit (unless they have research grants) that it's not going well. The incidence of cancer has increased, the death rate from cancer has increased, and survival rates haven't changed much. In fact, cancer is still the second leading cause of death in America—some 500,000 deaths in 1989, the latest year for which firm numbers are available. Since cancer is essentially a disease of aging, we can expect the mortality figures to rise higher and higher as the baby-boomer generation continues to grow older.

This war has spawned an impressive array of cancer-fighting weapons, including surgery, radiation, and anticancer drugs. The sad truth is that these weapons have had no more than a limited impact even with earlier detection.

Why aren't our anticancer weapons doing the job? Partly because, strangely enough, cancer cells aren't all that different from normal cells. Cancer cells are simply antisocial, in that they don't know when to stop growing. Because they're biologically so similar to normal cells, cancer cells are hard to target. So that's a large part of the problem: most of the weapons we have now just aren't specific enough or sophisticated enough to tell the difference between normal cells and their cancerous cousins.

As a result, most of our anticancer weapons are actually crude, blunt instruments. Surgery can excise large, concentrated tumors, but it does nothing for the smaller colonies of cancer cells that can spread through the body and seed new tumors. Radiation kills cancer cells, but it can also kill healthy cells in the surrounding neighborhood—to say nothing of suppressing the immune system and making the patient sick. Anticancer drugs (chemotherapy) are powerful poisons, but since they're not especially specific to cancer cells, they in effect poison the entire system. (As one writer put it, these drugs amount to "flooding an entire golf course with raging pesticides just to get at one clump of ragweed.") Wolfgang Wrasidlo, director of drug development at the renowned Scripps Clinic in La Jolla, California, speaks for many scientists when he says, "Everybody knows that our present cancer drugs are lousy."

Virtually all the experts acknowledge that a preferred way to treat cancer would be to enlist the patient's own body to fight off the disease. The human body is uniquely designed to defeat cancer, using the potent weaponry in its own immune system. (In fact, cancer can be defined as an immune-deficiency disease, a disease in which the immune system's weapons have been compromised or incapacitated.) With cancer, somehow the immune system has been short-circuited, and this enables the cancer cells not only to grow but eventually to migrate to other sites in the body. Once the cancer has migrated, or *metastasized*, the game is essentially over.

That's why some of the newest and most promising cancer treatments focus on getting the patient's immune system cranked up to attack the cancer—to attack it with far greater precision than any drug, radiation, or surgery. Medically, this approach is known as development of biological response modifiers. That means using bioengineered proteins to act as molecular bugles, calling the immune system to take action.

These bioengineered proteins—interferons, interleukin II, and tumor necrosis factor, for example—stimulate a platoon of immune-system cells, known as natural killer (NK) cells. NK cells are like heat-seeking missiles, relentlessly searching out cancer cells, homing on them, and destroying them.

In theory, this sounds good: use engineered proteins to muster the troops and fire the missiles. Still, up to now the results of this type of therapy, while somewhat encouraging, are far from spectacular.

In my view, it's because these therapies have essentially ignored the immune system's most important biological response modifier: eicosanoids. Cancer, like heart disease, can be understood as a condition in which eicosanoids are out of balance. I believe the ultimate strategy for fighting cancer is one that allows the body to prevent an overproduction of bad eicosanoids, which depress the immune system.

EICOSANOIDS AND CANCER

Since the mid-1980s, scientific research has shown that eicosanoids play a powerful role in the development of cancer. Bad eicosanoids, as you might imagine, are the villains of the piece, and there's a whole troop of them. PGE_2 suppresses the immune system by inhibiting the activation of NK cells so that they can't fight off cancers. Another group of bad eicosanoids, known as *lipoxins*, also inhibits the action of NK cells.

Other bad eicosanoids known as leukotrienes help cancer tumors sprout the new blood vessels they need to keep them nourished and growing. (This process is known as *angiogenesis*.) Meanwhile, yet another class of bad eicosanoids known as *hydroxylated essential fatty acids* actually promote metastasis—the potentially lethal tendency of cancers to spread throughout the body.

Unlike heart disease, in which both good and bad eicosanoids play a role, cancer appears to be the result of a runaway production of bad eicosanoids. So the goal in treating and preventing cancer is to clamp down on the synthesis of bad eicosanoids by choking off the supply of arachidonic acid.

To demonstrate the relationship between the overproduction of arachidonic acid and cancer I did a small pilot study of my own, using excised tumors from a variety of human cancers. I ground up the tumors, extracted the fatty acids, and analyzed them for their activated essential fatty acid content. (Remember that among the activated essential fatty acids, good eicosanoids are made from DGLA, while arachidonic acid is the building block for bad eicosanoids. So the balance of DGLA to arachidonic acid in a cancer cell may be the most important factor in determining a successful outcome.)

The results are shown below.

As you can see, the more aggressive the tumor, the lower its ratio of DGLA to arachidonic acid. (Pancreatic cancer tumors are among the most aggressive known.) This means that the more aggressive the tumor, the greater the potential to produce more bad eicosanoids.

Think of it this way: virtually all cancers develop a unique stealth strategy system to make their presence invisible to the immune system. How? By generating an overproduction of bad eicosanoids from

TABLE 14-1

DGLA to Arachidonic Acid in Various Human Tumors

TUMOR	DGLA/ARACHIDONIC ACID
Benign breast (n=4)	0.69 ± 0.24
Malignant breast (n=5)	0.34 ± 0.09
Colon (n=3)	0.19 ± 0.05
Pancreatic (n=1)	0.09

arachidonic acid. This gives a cancer cell an extraordinary means of self-protection, as well as a means to grow uncontrollably.

It follows, then, that tilting the body's eicosanoid balance away from bad eicosanoids should have a considerable positive impact on the cancer process. We tilt that balance using the most powerful drug known to man: food.

DIET AND CANCER

The existing treatments for cancer are probably the most barbaric in modern medicine. Faced with these blunt instruments, many cancer victims search desperately for alternative treatments, often turning to diet in the hope that changing what they eat will magically treat their disease. There are numerous Aunt Millie stories about how this diet or that diet cured cancer, but for most scientists those stories are easy to dismiss.

Rather than dismiss them, though, I always try to find a kernel of truth, something that makes hormonal sense, and that may be applicable to a wider population.

Take macrobiotics, for example. In the cancer-patient "underground," macrobiotics have attracted a considerable following, and generated an impressive number of Aunt Millie stories. But there does seem to be some science behind these claims. In 1993, for example, the *Journal of the American College of Nutrition* published a study on the use of a macrobiotic diet in cancer treatment. In this study, using patients with pancreatic cancer, 52 percent of those who followed a macrobiotic diet were still alive after one year, compared to only 10 percent of those who made no dietary changes. In other words, the macrobiotic diet was producing a 500 percent increase in one-year survival rates.

If you put aside all the New Age philosophy that often accompanies macrobiotic diets, you can see it clearly in terms of its ability to modulate eicosanoids. First, the macrobiotic diet is low in total fat, so it chokes off supplies of omega 6 essential fatty acids. In that way it meets the first criterion for a sound anticancer diet: low total fat intake. Low total fat—especially omega 6 fatty acids—means less arachidonic acid, and fewer bad eicosanoids.

Second, the macrobiotic diet is rich in the activated omega 3 essential fatty acid, EPA. That's because the macrobiotic diet emphasizes fish and sea vegetables, which are extraordinarily rich in EPA. Now, sea vegetables are not common items in Western diets, nor are they very appetizing to the Western palate. Even so, macrobiotic diets meet the second criterion for a sound anticancer diet—a rich EPA content. Ultimately, this means that the body's production of arachidonic acid is restricted even further.

In terms of eicosanoid balance, then, the macrobiotic diet looks good, in that it limits the supplies for making bad eicosanoids. Unfortunately, it's also rich in unfavorable carbohydrates, especially grains. You'll remember that unfavorable carbohydrates increase levels of insulin, and that means more bad eicosanoids. So this violates the third criteria for a sound anticancer diet—reduction of insulin levels—and thereby limits many of the macrobiotic diet's potential eicosanoid benefits.

It's like taking two steps forward and one step back. Some progress, but not nearly enough—especially if one has cancer.

All right, if the macrobiotic diet doesn't quite fit the bill for an anticancer diet, what about vegetarian diets? Well, strict vegetarian diets are low in total fats, and that can mean fewer bad eicosanoids simply because of the decrease in omega 6 fatty-acid intake. But that's counterbalanced by an excessive amount of carbohydrates, meaning more insulin and more bad eicosanoids. At the same time, strict vegetarian diets have very limited amounts of EPA (if any), so that they have a limited capacity to inhibit the formation of arachidonic acid.

In the end, then, the vegetarian diet is like one step forward and two steps backward. So, for the cancer patient, it's actually less desirable than a macrobiotic diet.

Finally, there's the American Cancer Society diet. This diet invariably fails for the same reasons that the American Heart Association diet fails. They're both too high in carbohydrates, so they both induce excessively high insulin levels. At the same time, the absolute levels of fat—and therefore omega 6 fatty acids—are too high. That means too much arachidonic acid and too many bad eicosanoids. Bad news for the heart patient, and especially bad news for the cancer patient.

DIET AND CANCER: THE ANIMAL MODELS

Macrobiotics, vegetarian diets, the American Cancer Society diet—all these have been used for years in an attempt to prevent and treat cancer in humans, at best meeting with limited success. In animals, however, there are two dietary approaches that have consistently been shown to have dramatic anticancer effects.

One of those approaches is simply to restrict calories. I'll explore the effect of calorie restriction on overall life extension in greater detail in a later chapter, but for now I'll just say that in animals, at least, *calorie restriction—coupled with the correct macronutrient composition—is far more effective than any drug in the prevention or treatment of cancer.*

There are two mechanisms by which calorie restriction positively affects cancer. First, calorie restriction reduces insulin levels, and in doing so decreases the overproduction of bad eicosanoids that promote tumor growth. Second, since total calories are reduced in these diets, so are total fats. As in any low-fat diet, this in turn decreases the intake of saturated fat that can possibly lead to insulin resistance. At the same time, reduction in fat limits the supply of the omega 6 fatty acids that can potentially be made into bad eicosanoids.

Caloric restriction is not the only dietary approach that has helped fight cancer in animals. An equally successful technique involves feeding the animals high levels of fish oils rich in EPA. Why is this approach effective? Because EPA limits activity of the enzyme delta 5 desaturase, which converts DGLA (the building block of good eicosanoids) into arachidonic acid (the building block of bad eicosanoids). More EPA, less delta 5 desaturase activity. Less delta 5 desaturase activity, less production of arachidonic acid. Less arachidonic acid, fewer bad eicosanoids. Cutting down on the production of bad eicosanoids is the secret of preventing, if not reversing, cancer in animals.

I firmly believe that the ideal diet for the cancer patient would be a diet that minimizes the production of bad eicosanoids by reducing levels of arachidonic acid. Such a diet would have four important features: it would be low in total fat content (thereby reducing both saturated fat and linoleic-acid intake) and rich in EPA; have adequate protein to prevent muscle wasting; and control the balance of good and bad eicosanoids by maintaining the appropriate protein-to-carbohydrate ratio at every meal.

What diet does all this? You already know the answer. A Zone-favorable diet. However, there are a few differences, though, between the Zone-favorable diet that most people can follow and the version that's designed specifically for the cancer patient. The cancer patient should:

1. Completely eliminate red meat, egg yolks, and organ meats from the diet. (This is also a requirement in the macrobiotic diet.)
2. Reduce intake of omega 6 essential fatty acid to very low levels. (Again, this is similar to the macrobiotic diet.)
3. Make sure that most of the fat in the diet is coming from monounsaturated fat and fish oil, with salmon as the primary fish source of EPA. (This is similar to the macrobiotic diet, but without the use of exotic sea vegetables.)
4. Add extra EPA in the form of dietary fish-oil supplements. The fish oil should be molecularly distilled. A reasonable amount would be an extra 1,000 mg of EPA per day. (This is in line with the macrobiotic diet.)
5. Restrict total calorie intake, but ensure protein adequate to prevent loss of lean body mass.
6. Maintain a strict ratio of three grams of protein for every four grams of carbohydrate at every meal.
7. Make sure that most of the carbohydrates eaten come from fruits or fiber-rich vegetables.

Obviously, in terms of treating cancer the Zone-favorable diet and the macrobiotic diet have a lot in common. But the Zone-favorable diet should do a much better job in limiting the production of arachidonic acid, and therefore reducing bad eicosanoid formation. Besides, it's a lot easier to comply with. For any cancer patient, a Zone-favorable diet should be your first line of defense.

Although this is an Aunt Millie story, it's still highly suggestive, in that it shows the power of a Zone-favorable diet in fighting one of the most dangerous of all cancers: brain tumors. In July of 1993, Judy Jones was stricken with a seizure that was initially thought to be a stroke. Six months later, tests revealed that in fact Judy was suffering from two different brain tumors, one growing on top of the other. In December of 1993, a biopsy indicated that both tumors were malignant. Emergency surgery removed one of the tumors, but only part of the other.

Needless to say, that Christmas was not a joyous one for Judy. For the next six weeks she had radiation treatments, even though most cancer specialists would not expect much success at such a late stage. She also did something else. In January, she started following a Zone-favorable diet.

In April, when her radiation treatments were finished, Judy had a magnetic resonance imaging (MRI) scan so that her doctors could begin to track the eventual growth of her remaining tumor. Her next MRI brain scan, six months later, left her doctors shaking their heads in astonishment. The tumor was not only shrinking, it appeared to be dead—a highly unexpected, if not unheard-of result. All the doctors could say was "Come back next year."

For Judy, Christmas in 1994 was a little different from the year before. During the week before Christmas, she worked fifty-six hours to give her coworkers time off for their shopping. Judy told me that she hadn't felt this good in five years.

Living in the Zone is the best revenge against cancer.

BREAST CANCER, DIET, AND THE ZONE

Although far more women will die of heart disease, the greatest fear for most women remains breast cancer. From a scientific point of view, breast cancer gives a unique insight into how the diet affects the course of cancer in general.

There is a body of evidence which suggests that eating a high-fat diet increases the risk of breast cancer. Remember: when you eat more fat, you also eat more linoleic acid. If that increased linoleic acid is driven primarily toward arachidonic acid, you can expect an overall depression of the immune system. That can spell cancer, including breast cancer.

Hold on, though. A 1994 study in the *Journal of the American Medical Association* reported that there is no association between dietary fat and breast cancer. In the same year a study in the *New England Journal of Medicine* indicated that it's not the amount of fat women eat that determines the likelihood of developing breast cancer, but how fat they are. In fact, in predicting the likelihood of breast cancer, obesity turns out to be an even greater risk factor than a prior family history of breast cancer. The effect of obesity on breast cancer should be one of the greatest fears of the medical establishment. Like men, women in this country are getting fatter and fatter. This means that their risk for breast cancer is increasing like a ticking time bomb.

You now know that obesity means elevated insulin levels. That in turn means a chronic oversupply of bad eicosanoids, and too many bad eicosanoids decrease the cancer-fighting efficiency of the immune system.

Elevated insulin levels have an even more insidious effect: they bring on a corresponding reduction in the circulating amounts of the vital proteins that bind sex hormones, especially estrogen. These proteins act as a biological drug-delivery system, latching onto free estrogen so that it can't bind to estrogen receptors in the breast tissue. If the levels of these crucial proteins drop, then the estrogen can interact with abandon with the receptors on the breast tissue. That can stimulate the growth of potential breast cancer tumors.

What's the newest approach to preventing breast cancer? Giving high-risk patients a very powerful antitumor drug known as tamoxifen. Tamoxifen inhibits the binding of free estrogen to the receptor sites in the breast tissue.

I think there's a far better way to do this: raise the natural levels of the estrogen-binding proteins by reducing elevated insulin levels. This gives you a second weapon in the fight against breast cancer: if you reduce insulin levels, you reduce obesity. If you reduce obesity, you've dramatically reduced a major factor that puts you at risk of developing breast cancer in the first place.

CACHEXIA

There's a flip side to the story of diet and cancer. You see, cancer tumors are dietary hogs. They feed themselves by stealing nutrients from the rest of the body. As a result, the rest of the body slowly starves. This is known as wasting, or by its medical name, *cachexia*.

To make matters worse, many of our current cancer treatments compromise the gastrointestinal system's ability to absorb food. Result: malnutrition. In fact, it's estimated that *nearly 40 percent of all cancer patients don't die of cancer at all. They die of starvation, or of malnutrition induced by the treatments that were supposed to cure them.*

There should be an easy way to turn the tables. To the simpleminded (like me), it seems obvious that one useful dietary strategy for cancer treatment would be to starve the cancer, but not the rest of the body. But how? Well, it's known that cancer tumors grow best in an anaerobic environment (with a lack of oxygen), and thrive in the presence of high levels of carbohydrates. So you should be able to gag the tumors with a diet that increases the supply of oxygen and simultaneously starves them, depriving them of the carbohydrates they love. You do that by having cancer patients follow a Zone-favorable diet.

In the end, this simple, safe, and healthful strategy will not only help save cancer patients by eliminating cachexia and malnutrition, it will also restore the favorable balance of eicosanoids that is the best defense against cancer of all kinds, including breast cancer.

That's right: the best weapons in the war against cancer aren't pills or potions, or magic herbs, or gruesome anticancer treatments. The best cancer-fighting (and the best cancer-preventing) weapon is the food you put in your mouth.

CHAPTER FIFTEEN

CHRONIC DISEASES AND THE ZONE

Of all the maladies that lay people low, chronic diseases can be among the most frustrating, to the point of terror. Once they're lodged in the body, these diseases simply don't go away, no matter how many pills you take, no matter how many doctors (or psychiatrists) you visit, no matter how much money you spend. They're like a life sentence with no possibility of parole, and no time off for good behavior.

I've come to think of many of these chronic diseases as either/or conditions: either you can treat them—or at least reduce their severity—by using a Zone-favorable diet, or there's no treatment that's effective in the long run. You see, virtually every disease—including many of the chronic diseases—can be understood in these terms of the Zone: the body is simply making too many bad eicosanoids and not enough good ones. If that's true, then a Zone-favorable diet should be helpful in treating any or all of these diseases.

I realize that those are bold and sweeping statements, but there are very strong scientific indications to back them up. First of all, there are clinical studies which show that many chronic diseases have responded to dietary supplementation with activated essential fatty acids (EPA and GLA)—the same essential fatty acids that I was using in my earlier work to reach the Zone, the same essential fatty acids that are critical to regulate eicosanoid balance. At the same time, there's evidence in the scientific literature that for some chronic diseases direct injections of good eicosanoids such as PGE_1 have clinical benefits.

Finally, there's a wealth of studies that show the effectiveness of aspirin, nonsteroidal anti-inflammatory drugs (NSAIDs), and corticosteroids—all drugs that suppress the overproduction of bad eicosanoids. All this evidence supports my contention that these chronic diseases should be viewed as eicosanoid-disturbance conditions, and as such would benefit from a Zone-favorable diet.

Here are some of the chronic diseases that can be attacked with a Zone-favorable diet. It's a long list, and some of them will surprise you.

AIDS

If we've been losing the war on cancer, then the battle against AIDS has been an utter and shameful defeat. At the moment, we really have only one anti-AIDS drug—AZT—and the 1994 International AIDS conference in Tokyo sadly confirmed that AZT doesn't necessarily prolong the lives of AIDS victims. Sadder still, the outlook for future breakthroughs is not optimistic. In fact, the next International Conference on AIDS will be held in 1996, instead of 1995, in hopes that in the ensuing two years some new drug or vaccine will have been discovered.

The real problem here is that billions of research dollars have been invested in treating AIDS as a purely viral disease, yet results from this approach have been lacking. Is it possible that AIDS is *not* simply a viral disease?

In the early stages of the AIDS epidemic, there was a massive rush among the experts (many of whom were veterans of the war on cancer) to reach a consensus as to what might be the cause of AIDS, and therefore the "appropriate" treatment. The experts settled on the notion of infection by a single virus as the most likely explanation. Robert Root-Bernstein, a professor at Michigan State University and leading critic of the current thinking on AIDS, points out in his seminal book *Rethinking AIDS* that this notion has led the AIDS research community down a dead-end path. *Rethinking AIDS* asks one central and crucial question: "Is it possible that other approaches that might provide an effective way to treat AIDS were crowded out in the early rush to reach a scientific consensus?"

As early as 1984, I became convinced that AIDS could be viewed as an eicosanoid-imbalance disease. Actually, the clues had been around since the 1950s.

The clinical definition of AIDS is the appearance of opportunistic infections—parasitic, fungus, or viral infections that are easily fought off when the immune system is functioning normally. Many of these opportunistic infections first appeared in the 1950s with the advent of the newest wonder drugs: corticosteroids. There was virtually no disease state that did not initially show a dramatic improvement with the use of corticosteroids, like cortisone and prednisone. But if patients continued taking these drugs for more than thirty days, their immune systems virtually stopped working.

What happened? They developed opportunistic infections similar to those that we now see in people with AIDS—the same types of infections that a reasonably active immune system easily repels. (By the way, they're also the same types of infections that commonly occur in cancer patients undergoing chemotherapy, which also depresses the immune system.)

In the 1970s the work of Anthony Fauci (now head of AIDS research at the National Institutes of Health) provided another clue. Fauci showed that a single injection of corticosteroids into normal volunteers dramatically reduced the number of T-cells—particularly T-helper cells, the same kind of immune cells that are disabled in AIDS. So corticosteroids were producing (temporarily, at least) a condition that looked very much like AIDS.

How do corticosteroids work in the body? They're like super-aspirins: they knock out all eicosanoid synthesis, and they knock it out for long periods of time. (Aspirin only knocks out a subgroup of eicosanoids, prostaglandins, and only for short periods of time.) Could the HIV virus be acting like the corticosteroids—as a massive inhibitor of all eicosanoid synthesis? I thought so.

There are other viruses that have been shown to inhibit the delta 6 desaturase enzyme, thereby shutting down the production of essential fatty acids and eicosanoids. To me it seemed likely that HIV may have the same effect, but with much more power. That effect on essential fatty-acid metabolism would have the same consequences as continued long-term corticosteroid use: it would shut down all eicosanoid synthesis, and leave the immune system running on empty.

To me this sounded like a good hypothesis, but it needed testing. Fortunately, in 1988 I met two Pittsburgh physicians, Paul Kahl and Sam Golden, whose practice included a great number of patients infected with HIV. As clinicians faced with the stark reality of AIDS, Paul and Sam were aware that the drugs promoted by the research establishment were not particularly effective where it counted—in people actually infected with HIV.

Luckily, Paul had completed his medical training at New York

University, which was a hotbed of early eicosanoid research. Like many physicians with a bit of knowledge of eicosanoids, Paul knew all about bad eicosanoids, but never knew there might be good ones as well. Intrigued by the possibility that a purely dietary program could help people with HIV infection who were suffering from chronic fatigue—induced either by the infection itself or by high doses of AZT—we organized a double-blind, placebo-controlled study using patients with ARC (AIDS-Related Complex).

In this study we used either combinations of activated essential fatty acids containing EPA and GLA or a placebo (olive oil) for two different groups of Paul and Sam's patients: one group of people infected with HIV and suffering chronic fatigue, but not taking AZT; and the other group of HIV-infected patients who were taking high doses of AZT (1,500 mg per day). We randomly assigned these patients to take either the activated essential fatty acids or the placebo.

Since I had not yet understood the importance of controlling the insulin-to-glucagon ratio, in this study we were using a less sophisticated approach: trying to move the patients into the Zone simply by using activated essential fatty acids alone.

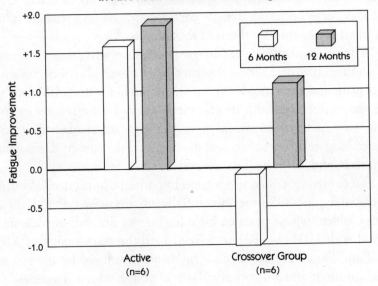

Effects of Activated Essential Fatty Acids in ARC Patients with Chronic Fatigue

Figure 15-1

After six months, we found that the patients on the activated essential fatty-acid supplements were dramatically less fatigued than the patients who took only the placebo. These results are shown in Figure 15-1 and in Table 15-1. Fatigue improvement was based on physician assessment, on a five-point scale, from –2 (significantly increased fatigue) to +2 (significantly decreased fatigue), with a score of zero meaning no change in fatigue.

The differences between the groups of patients not taking AZT were statistically significant, at a p factor of less than 0.005. This means that we were confident that if 1,000 HIV-infected patients with chronic fatigue supplemented their diets with the same combinations of activated essential fatty acids, then we could expect that 995 would see some alleviation of fatigue. In those patients taking high doses of AZT (1,500 mg per day), we saw essentially the same results, although with a lower p factor of 0.025. This meant we were confident that 97 out of 100 HIV patients taking high doses of AZT were likely to see alleviation of their fatigue with supplementation of activated essential fatty acids.

This improvement took place in spite of the fact that during the six months the number of T-helper cells—the cells that are killed by HIV—were dropping faster in the active group than in the placebo group. This seems paradoxical, but still, the patients were improving, especially the patients who were taking AZT. In the placebo group, T-cell counts were not dropping, and yet these patients were increasingly fatigued. Actually, it's not such a surprising paradox; any AIDS clinician can tell you that many patients with relatively high T-helper cell counts die of AIDS, whereas many with low T-helper cells survive. In fact, we had one patient whose T-cell count was extremely low (less than 10), but who played tennis every day.

Encouraged by the alleviation of fatigue, we switched the patients on the placebo olive-oil capsules to the capsules containing the same combinations of activated essential fatty acids as those in the active group. At the same time, we kept the original group on activated essential fatty acids for another six months. The results were the same: a significant alleviation of fatigue.

The original group with chronic fatigue (but not taking AZT), who supplemented with activated essential fatty acids, continued to improve. More important, the group that had been switched from the

TABLE 15-1

Effect of Activated Essential Fatty-Acid Combinations on HIV-Infected Patients with Chronic Fatigue

PARAMETER	ACTIVE GROUP	PLACEBO GROUP	SIGNIFICANCE
Patients not taking AZT	(n=6)	(n=6)	
Fatigue assessment at 6 months	+1.5	–1.0	P < 0.005
Change in T4 cells	–30%	–14%	P < 0.01
Patients taking AZT	(n=5)	(n=4)	
Fatigue assessment at 6 months	+1.0	–0.5	P < 0.025
Change in T4 cells	–58%	0%	P > 0.025

placebo to activated essential fatty acids now showed a complete reversal in their fatigue pattern, with a p factor of less than 0.01, meaning we were confident that 99 out of 100 patients would see reversal of their fatigue. These were almost exactly the same results we initially got with the original group. For those patients taking AZT, there was also a reversal of fatigue, but the results were not statistically significant (owing simply to the fact that we were working with a limited number of patients). These results are shown in Table 15-2, and graphically in Figure 15-2.

You can imagine our excitement. This was the only double-blind, placebo-controlled, crossover study ever done in AIDS research—even though we funded it out of our own pockets.

Next, we did what any good scientist would do: we presented our results in the appropriate forum—in this case the Fifth International AIDS Conference at Montreal in 1989. Unfortunately, we received a

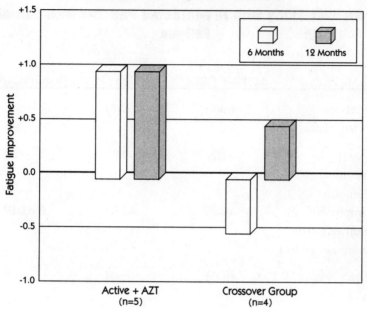

Figure 15-2

very lukewarm reception. The AIDS research community seemed to view our work as little more than a health-food gimmick—not good science like their work with AZT. And who needed diet when it was clear (to them, at least) that AZT was going to eradicate the AIDS epidemic?

But we weren't flying solo. A year after we presented our initial results at the AIDS conference in Montreal, another investigator, Terry Pulse, published similar data using slightly different combinations of EPA and GLA. Unfortunately, he published his work in a rather obscure journal, so it languished in much the same way as Craven's work on aspirin. Although Pulse's work confirmed the results of our pilot study in terms of improving the quality of life of patients infected with HIV, both these pieces of the AIDS puzzle were lost in the din of the victory chants for AZT.

Five years later AIDS is still going strong, and the scientific honeymoon with AZT is over. This wasn't surprising to me. I knew that the National Cancer Institute had stopped all testing of AZT in can-

TABLE 15-2

Crossover Study with HIV-Infected Patients with Chronic Fatigue

PARAMETER	ACTIVE GROUP	PLACEBO GROUP	SIGNIFICANCE
Patients not taking AZT	(n=6)	(n=6)	
Fatigue assessment at 12 months	+1.7	+1.0	
Net improvement compared to 6-month assessment	+0.2	+2.0	P < 0.01
Patients taking AZT	(n=5)	(n=4)	
Fatigue assessment at 12 months	+1.0	+0.5	
Net improvement compared to 6-month assessment	0.0	+1.0	n.s.

cer patients ten years earlier because it proved to be too toxic for cancer patients. In fact, a decade earlier I had tried myself to reduce the toxicity of AZT, but without success.

Since the AIDS research community—and especially the funding agencies—were ignoring the potential for the dietary modulation of eicosanoids, I decided not to spend any more time or money (since I was funding my own research) on AIDS patients. I went back to my primary area of interest: treating cardiovascular patients.

By 1992 my research with cardiovascular patients was clearly showing that you could generate far better control of eicosanoids by controlling insulin and glucagon than you could with activated essential fatty-acid supplements alone. (Yes, HIV-infected patients would probably still need some activated essential fatty-acid supplementation, but only a fraction of the amount I had used in the 1989 pilot study.) Since I now had a more comprehensive approach for eicosanoid control, my interest in AIDS was renewed. At the same time, it had now become clear that AZT was no wonder drug.

In September of 1992, I got the chance to retest my theories on HIV infection when a friend asked me if there was anything I could do for Bill B. Bill (not his real name) was a successful Boston lawyer whose world began to unravel in 1988 when his doctors told him the grim news: blood tests showed that he was infected with HIV. Although he had not yet developed the full-blown disease, he was already suffering from chronic weakness, fever, and fatigue.

By March of 1991 Bill was so sick that he was forced to go on disability. Seven months later he was diagnosed with full-blown AIDS. His T-cell count was dropping rapidly and he had developed Karposi's sarcoma, a form of skin cancer that had been rare until AIDS came along. By September of 1992, his prognosis was poor.

I said I might be able to help, but only if Bill was willing to follow a two-pronged program, a program that included both a Zone-favorable diet and supplementation with activated essential fatty acids. I met with Bill, described the program's strategy for strengthening the immune system through eicosanoid control.

The last two years, since that first meeting, have been very good to Bill. He no longer suffers from fatigue. He works out five days a week. This past year he bought a thirty-foot sailboat, and he spent most of the summer sailing up and down the New England seacoast. And even though his T-cell counts remain low (about 30), since he started following a Zone-favorable diet over two years ago, he has not had a single opportunistic infection.

The word of Bill's striking success soon spread to a group of HIV patients who were members of the Boston Living Center, an AIDS support group. With Bill's help, we assembled a group of patients who were willing to follow a Zone-favorable diet. In 1994, the patients in the group saw results similar to Bill's, especially with regard to reduction of chronic fatigue. As long as they're in the Zone, they lead normal lives. As soon as they wander out of the Zone, life gets a lot tougher. So I remind them constantly that if they can *stay* in the

Zone, there's no reason they can't enjoy full and productive lives.

I think they're now believing it. Bill certainly does.

AUTOIMMUNE DISEASES

There are many researchers, including Robert Root-Bernstein, who think that AIDS is essentially an autoimmune disease, a disease in which the body's armies of defense—the immune system—turn traitor and attack the body itself. In the case of AIDS, the body may be attacking its own T-cells. (If this is so, then classical antiviral treatments, such as AZT, will never be successful.)

Let's take it one step further. All autoimmune diseases (potentially including AIDS) can be seen as diseases that result from an imbalance of eicosanoids. It's this imbalance—specifically the overproduction of bad eicosanoids—that causes the body to attack itself, to develop the hair-trigger immune response that defines autoimmunity.

There are a great many autoimmune diseases, but probably the most widespread is arthritis. Usually, arthritis is treated with anti-inflammatory drugs—aspirin, nonsteroidal anti-inflammatory drugs (NSAID's), or corticosteroids. All these anti-inflammatories have the same mode of action. They all stop eicosanoid production, good and bad. Their only differences lie in their relative ability to stop eicosanoid formation. Corticosteroids are the most powerful, but they're also the most dangerous, since they shut down eicosanoid production so thoroughly that the immune system shuts down as well.

Well, if arthritis is a result of eicosanoid imbalance, then the eicosanoid-modulating benefits of a Zone-favorable diet should definitely help arthritis sufferers.

How do I know? Numerous clinical studies have shown that dietary supplementation with activated essential fatty acids—GLA and EPA, either singly or in combination—reduces arthritic pain and inflammation. If you get positive results with supplements of activated essential fatty acids, that's a strong indication that a Zone-favorable diet (designed to maintain a favorable balance of eicosanoids) would do the job just as well or better.

A Zone-favorable diet should be the first line of defense in the treatment of arthritis. In fact, the more closely an arthritic patient follows a Zone-favorable diet, the fewer anti-inflammatory drugs he or she should need to control pain. On the other hand, the further from the Zone the diet takes the arthritic patient, the more that patient will need those anti-inflammatory drugs to slow down an increasing production of pro-inflammatory eicosanoids.

The choice seems simple. While a Zone-favorable diet may never totally eliminate the need for anti-inflammatory drugs, anything that can reduce the amount of medication will be of long-term benefit for arthritis sufferers.

A Zone-favorable diet is a safe and effective frontal assault on arthritis pain and inflammation. But the diet has an important and positive side effect as well: loss of excess body fat. Because it decreases the load on weight-bearing joints like the knees, losing body fat can only aid the reduction of arthritic pain.

Although arthritis may be the most common autoimmune disease, the most terrifying is multiple sclerosis (MS). Unlike arthritis, in which the body is attacking the tissue in the joints, in MS the body attacks the fatty insulation layer (called the myelin sheath) that surrounds the nerves in the central nervous system. When that insulation unravels, nerve conduction is slowed, and as a result there's a subsequent loss of muscle control.

You can view MS as arthritis inside the central nervous system. So you'd think that the same drugs that are effective in treating arthritis should also be effective in treating MS. They're not. To treat a disease of the central nervous system, a drug must be able to reach the brain. Anti-inflammatory drugs can't do that because they're water-soluble, and the brain has a unique membrane, known as the blood-brain barrier, that prevents virtually all water-soluble drugs from entering.

Essential fatty acids and eicosanoids are fats. They have no trouble at all getting through the blood-brain barrier. In fact, the brain itself is mostly composed of fat, which is also the prime structural component of the myelin membrane.

All right: if MS results from inflammation of the myelin sheath, you'd think it would be possible to reduce that inflammation by reducing the amount of pro-inflammatory bad eicosanoids while simultaneously increasing the amount of anti-inflammatory good eicosa-noids. How do you do that? With a Zone-favorable diet.

This is exactly what happens with MS patients on a Zone-favor-able diet. Just as with HIV-infected patients, one of the immediate benefits is a significant reduction in fatigue. Some cases in point: Dr. Paul Kahl, the same physician with whom I did the AIDS pilot study, told me the story of one of his patients, a fifty-year-old woman with MS. Paul put her on a Zone-favorable diet, and after a few months on the program she came in for a checkup. Paul asked the basic question: "How are your feeling?" Her answer was "Great!" Noticing that she was still using a cane for stability, Paul asked her, "If you're feeling so great, why are you still using the cane?" Her only response was that since developing MS she always had.

Paul took the cane away and told her to walk to the end of the hallway and back. After a few tentative steps, she made the round trip quickly. When Paul asked her if she wanted her cane back, she just smiled and told him to keep it for someone who really needed it.

Then there's the case of Phoebe Stark, who had what is known as progressive chronic MS. In this phase of the disease, the patient be-comes progressively weaker, so that completing simple daily tasks is terribly fatiguing. Phoebe started on a Zone-favorable diet, and within a month she remarked, "I can finally live again." Although she had some slight residual effects of MS, the quality of her life has dra-matically improved.

I'm the first to admit that these stories are not unlike the typical testimonials that you'd expect to hear at a faith-healing revival meet-ing. I tell them because they strongly suggest that in an autoimmune disease like MS—a disease that has a significant inflammatory com-ponent—a Zone-favorable diet can provide a significant benefit sim-ply by changing eicosanoid levels.

There's actually a lot of good science to support this notion. For example, recent research shows that chronic progressive MS patients have higher levels of PGE_2 in their blood than normal people or pa-tients with stable MS. Also, just prior to MS attacks, levels of PGE_2 are elevated. Other research has shown increased levels of leuko-trienes in the cerebrospinal fluid of MS patients. Since PGE_2 and leukotrienes are pro-inflammatory eicosanoids, any reduction in their levels would be consistent with the benefits reported by MS pa-tients following a Zone-favorable diet.

There's more. Over the past thirty years, the work of Roy Swank has indicated that a diet low in saturated fat is beneficial for MS patients. Since a Zone-favorable diet is designed to limit saturated fat, Swank's observations are also consistent with the benefits reported by our patients.

The newest breakthrough in MS treatment involves injections of interferons, substances that help regulate the immune system. Since bad eicosanoids like PGE_2 inhibit the release of interferons, any reduction in PGE_2 levels would be likely to rev up the body's natural production of interferons. And, of course, a Zone-favorable diet limits PGE_2 production.

Put all this together, and you come to one conclusion: a Zone-favorable diet is a reasonable diet for any MS patient at any stage of the disease.

Another autoimmune disease in which modulation of eicosanoid levels has been found effective—in animals, at least—is lupus. Animal models of lupus can be developed by the selected inbreeding of mice. These animals will all die of lupus within a year. Yet studies at the University of Pennsylvania have shown that if these same inbred animals are injected with PGE_1 (one of the good eicosanoids), they'll live.

All this is strong evidence that a Zone-favorable diet can be of benefit in treating any type of autoimmune disease, whether it's AIDS, arthritis, multiple sclerosis, or lupus. In the Zone, all these diseases will improve, simply because a Zone-favorable diet reduces the overproduction of bad eicosanoids and increases the production of good eicosanoids—a combination that's ideal for treating the inflammatory conditions generated by autoimmune diseases.

How much improvement can patients with autoimmune diseases expect? Using the diet alone, it's variable. It appears that autoimmune diseases cause residual defects in the body's ability to make activated essential fatty acids. So in addition to following a Zone-favorable diet very closely, these patients will require small amounts of activated essential fatty-acid supplements to help them stay in the Zone.

All this makes exquisite good sense. After all, an appropriate diet coupled with the least amount of drug required to control a disease is simply good medicine.

CHRONIC FATIGUE

For a patient with an autoimmune disease, the greatest improvement in quality of life is the alleviation of fatigue. Can a Zone-favorable diet benefit patients with fatigue that's caused by viral infections—or even fatigue that seems to have no known cause? Again, the answer appears to be yes.

I believe that a great number of fatigue-related conditions may start with some type of viral infection. This is strongly suggested with arthritis and multiple sclerosis, although the culprit viruses have not yet been isolated. Obviously in AIDS, the HIV virus is the underlying factor that brings on fatigue. Chronic fatigue syndrome (CFS) is still another disease characterized by fatigue in which a viral origin seems to be implicated.

So there seems to be a link between viruses, long-lasting fatigue, activated essential fatty acids, and eicosanoids. Studies conducted at Ohio State University, for example, show that patients with chronic fatigue after mononucleosis (a viral infection) have a long-lasting defect in the body's ability to make GLA—and therefore all eicosanoids.

In another clinical study done at the University of Glasgow, patients with postviral fatigue syndrome who were given supplements of activated essential fatty acids had a statistically significant reduction in their fatigue compared to controls who were given placebo capsules. This report, which was very similar to our own work with HIV patients, is strongly suggestive that fatigue, when it stems from a viral infection, may simply be a consequence of being out of the Zone for a long period of time.

Think about the flu and how tired it makes you feel. Chronic fatigue is like having the flu all the time. The body has some reserve capacity to fight the eicosanoid damage brought on by a viral infection, but that capacity is not infinite. Once this reserve capacity for making eicosanoids is exhausted, fatigue sets in. That fatigue will continue unless something (a new medication, change in diet, or plain old good luck) intervenes to change the situation.

Since fatigue appears to be related to viral infections, small doses of activated essential fatty acids may be required in addition to following a Zone-favorable diet. Remember: supplements of these fatty acids are a relatively quick way to enter the Zone. But if you use activated essential fatty acids alone, the boundaries of the Zone will constantly shift. So unless you're following a Zone-favorable diet at the same time, you'll have to continually readjust your ratios and amounts of activated essential fatty acids. With a Zone-favorable diet the boundaries of the Zone are far more static and defined, so you'll need only small and occasional readjustments in the amounts of activated essential fatty acids to remain there on a continual basis.

A case in point is one of my neighbors, a noted physical therapist in the Boston area. About two years ago, I saw him walking around the block, which was unusual, since he was a marathon runner. He also seemed to be breathing heavily. Being neighborly, I asked him how he was doing. His answer was: "Terrible."

He told me that for the last six months he'd been experiencing the most intense fatigue imaginable. He couldn't stay awake during seminars, and he would fall asleep behind the wheel of his car if he drove for more than forty-five minutes. Basically, his life was rotten. He had taken every possible test known, but the best the Boston medical establishment could determine was that his cholesterol was slightly elevated.

I told him it sounded like a case of chronic fatigue, which none of his doctors had ever mentioned to him. I went inside my house and gave him some of the experimental bars I was using for my diabetic patients, some capsules containing the activated essential fatty acids, and several Zone-favorable meal plans to follow. I told him that if he followed this regimen in a week his fatigue would be significantly reduced.

He looked at me the same way that Jack's mother must have looked at Jack when he brought back the magic beans he got for selling the family's cow. But he said he was so desperate that no matter how stupid this sounded he'd try it.

Four days later he came back and said it might all be in his head, but he seemed to be a lot more active. A week later he took his family for a week at Disney World and was running circles around the kids. In fact, when the kids were ready to go back to the hotel and collapse, my neighbor had to beg them to go with him on one more ride. So much for chronic fatigue.

CENTRAL NERVOUS SYSTEM DISORDERS

The brain, as I mentioned earlier, is mostly fat. It's also exceptionally rich in essential fatty acids. So it should come as no surprise that a number of diseases of the central nervous system may be related to disturbances in eicosanoid balance.

Probably the most widely studied of these diseases is alcoholism. Alcohol is a fascinating drug with a long history. It's been around for some eight thousand years, making it older than many of the civilizations of man.

In small amounts, alcohol is a boon to the cardiovascular system. It increases the production of the good eicosanoids, which enhance cardiovascular function. But as we all know, alcohol has a dangerous dark side as well, one of the most dangerous of which is alcoholism. It's estimated that there are more than twenty million alcoholics in this country, and the negative impact of alcoholism on mortality, health-care costs, and social order is well known. Of course, not everyone who sips a beer after work or has a few cocktails at a party becomes an alcoholic. But at the same time, alcoholism is not a disease that strikes only the weak of will. There are many otherwise highly successful and disciplined people who seem to have absolutely no ability to control their alcohol intake. The truth is that alcoholism has a very strong genetic link, suggesting that there may be a genetic predisposition to the disease.

What is that link? It turns out that alcoholics have a genetic defect in making GLA, which ultimately means that their bodies' ability to make good eicosanoids is compromised. (In fact, blood levels of GLA in alcoholics are only 50 percent that of normal people.)

For most people, alcohol in moderate amounts actually speeds up the process of making good eicosanoids—for a while, at least. This explains both the long-term cardiovascular and short-term emotional benefits (good eicosanoids have an antidepressive activity) of moderate drinking.

Unfortunately, in people who have a genetic defect in making GLA, alcohol inhibits the normal replenishment of this activated essential fatty acid. And this sets up a vicious circle: the victims of alcoholism are depleting their limited reservoir of GLA, and at the same time preventing its replenishment. The unhappy result: to make good eicosanoids, the alcoholic needs more alcohol—just to feel normal.

Ask any ex-alcoholics—they'll tell you that even after many years of abstinence it's a constant struggle to stay alcohol-free. Yet when I began to work with recovering alcoholics using a Zone-favorable diet, the first thing they seemed to notice was that their craving for alcohol was greatly reduced, if not completely eliminated.

What's the biology behind this happy result? One immediate consequence of a Zone-favorable diet is that the activity of the delta 6 desaturase enzyme increases, and that means increased production of GLA. Once normal levels of GLA are reestablished, so is the normal production of good eicosanoids. So the underlying biological need for alcohol—as a drug to encourage eicosanoid formation—wanes.

In 1984, Ian Glen proved this in clinical trials with alcoholics, using GLA supplementation. By the end of the trial, the researchers noted a statistically significant reduction in alcohol cravings in these patients.

For the recovering alcoholic, being in the Zone means freedom from the biochemical defect that underlies alcoholism in the first place—a defect in eicosanoid metabolism. The prescription for achieving that freedom and maintaining it for life: low levels of activated essential fatty-acid supplementation coupled with a Zone-favorable diet.

Alcoholism isn't the only central-nervous-system disorder that responds to a Zone-favorable diet. Another is depression. Good eicosanoids have significant antidepressive effects because they increase the uptake and release of neurotransmitters from the nerves. (Neurotransmitters are the biochemical switches that allow one nerve to communicate with another.) If the levels of neurotransmitters drop (either by inhibition of their release from the transmitting nerve or their inhibition of uptake by the receiving nerve), the result is depression.

The current magic bullet for treating depression is the well-known drug Prozac. It increases the brain levels of a neurotransmitter called *serotonin*. With increased levels of serotonin, nerve communication is improved, and this alleviates depression.

Prozac works. It works so well that its sales are currently in the billions of dollars. But there's another way to treat depression without the expense and potential side effects of drugs—even effective drugs like Prozac.

What controls the release and uptake of neurotransmitters like serotonin? Good eicosanoids. By making more good eicosanoids, you're improving the effectiveness of neurological communication—whether you have depression or not. If you do suffer from depression—that is, from low levels of neurotransmitters—a Zone-favorable diet will increase the uptake and release of these vital chemical messengers, and that will help return you to normality.

Over the past few years, there's been a lot of attention paid, both from the media and in scientific circles, to another variety of depression: seasonal affective disorder, or SAD. In some people, as light cycles change with the onset of winter, the release of a hormone called *melatonin* from the pineal gland can become highly retarded. This melatonin deficiency can bring on SAD—more commonly known as the "winter blues."

Dr. Michael Norden, a research psychiatrist at the University of Washington Medical School, has been recommending a Zone-favorable diet to his SAD patients for the past two years. Michael tells me that a number of his patients report that the diet brings significant improvements. Increased production of good eicosanoids stimulate the release of melatonin in spite of the lowered light intensity of winter. If you've got the winter blues, a Zone-favorable diet might well make SADness a thing of the past.

While it may not qualify as depression (and, luckily, it's certainly not chronic), jet lag is SAD's biological cousin. Jet lag is the result of the readjustment of melatonin release in response to light-dark cycles that have changed too fast. So a Zone-favorable diet can help fight off jet lag, and maybe even wipe it out. (Personally, I used to have tremendous problems readjusting to East Coast time after traveling back from the West Coast. Now I actually look forward to cross-country traveling, because it gives me six hours of uninterrupted reading and writing time with no accompanying jet lag. Just another benefit of the Zone.)

If garden-variety depression stems from a sluggish neurotransmitter system, an overactive neurotransmitter system can bring on depression's behavioral opposite: extreme hyperactivity. Of course, simple hyperactivity can also be caused by low blood sugar. In either case, a Zone-favorable diet can help. If hyperactivity is a result of hypoglycemia (low blood sugar), then a Zone-favorable diet will help the body normalize blood-sugar levels. If overactive neurotransmitters are a problem, there's evidence that supplementation with activated essential fatty acids can help—especially for extremely hyperactive children. This suggests that a Zone-favorable diet might benefit these children as well.

But what if you're not depressed, or jet-lagged, or hyperactive? What if your levels of neurotransmitters are adequate, and your brain cells are hearing them loud and clear? A Zone-favorable diet will still provide valuable emotional rewards. Following a Zone-favorable diet will help you to handle the stresses and strains of everyday life with much greater ease. The stresses and strains won't change, but your central nervous system, bolstered by the increased production of good eicosanoids, will respond to those strains with aplomb, smoothing out your cruise down life's highway.

REPRODUCTIVE DISORDERS

Eicosanoids are intimately involved in the most complex biological control problem of them all: reproduction. Without eicosanoids, fertilization, and birth itself, would be impossible. So it's really not surprising that many reproductive disorders may have an eicosanoid imbalance as their underlying cause.

The best-documented connection between reproductive disorders and eicosanoids is every woman's (and every husband's) nightmare—premenstrual syndrome, or PMS.

Like alcoholism, PMS appears to be linked to a genetic defect in the normal synthesis of GLA. In fact, while alcoholics have GLA levels 50 percent lower than normal, the plasma levels of GLA in women suffering from PMS are estimated to be only 20 percent of normal.

Since the 1980s, a number of clinical studies have indicated that supplementation with activated essential fatty acids provides significant relief from PMS. There are other studies, however, that show no benefit from activated essential fatty-acid supplementation. I think these conflicting results are due to the fact that the boundaries of the

Zone tend to shift if you try to reach it through activated essential fatty-acid supplementation alone. To stabilize those shifting boundaries, it's essential to combine limited activated essential fatty-acid supplementation with a Zone-favorable diet.

That's what I've done in hundreds of PMS patients, and it works: these patients report significant reduction, if not eradication, of PMS within thirty to sixty days.

PMS might be a husband's nightmare, but what really terrifies most men is impotence. What's one of the most widely used treatments for impotence? Injections of a good eicosanoid, PGE_1, directly into the penis about thirty minutes prior to intercourse. What does the PGE_1 do? The same thing it does elsewhere in the body: it dramatically increases blood flow, and increased blood flow to the penis can spell erection.

Of course, injecting a syringe needle into the penis just before intercourse can be a real mood breaker. So why not take the easy, painless way to keep the blood supply flowing? A Zone-favorable diet will keep the body churning out the good eicosanoids—including PGE_1—that help maintain dilated blood vessels, and do it without turning the bedroom into an outpatient clinic.

Over the last four years I've received many reports from elderly men telling me that after about six months of being on a Zone-favorable diet their sexual performance improved dramatically. Of course, these are merely testimonials, not controlled scientific studies. Still, these happy men used no drugs, no injections, no magic aphrodisiacs. Just food.

CHRONIC PAIN

Everyone knows what pain feels like, but few people know the medical definition of chronic pain. From a doctor or a scientist's point of view, chronic pain is a persistent generation of the biochemical mediators of pain that travel via the nerves to the central nervous system.

There are usually two causes of chronic pain, and they usually coexist. The first is an actual structural impingement on the nerve fibers themselves. In other words, something's rubbing against the nerves and making them send pain signals to the brain. That something can be hard structural components like bones or disks (especially in the spine), or softer structural components like muscle. Obviously, unless the structural problem is taken care of, the pain will be constant.

Chiropractic treatment has evolved to make structural adjustments to relieve this kind of impingement on the nerves. The field of muscle therapy (myotherapy) can help to relieve pain caused by muscle impingement. The kind of massage you typically get in a health spa is a more limited and less defined way of affecting soft-tissue misalignment and the resulting pain. Still, this kind of massage usually does help people feel better—for a while, at least.

Since pain is difficult to quantify, claims for the effectiveness of chiropractic and muscle therapy remain unsupported, even though thousands of case studies suggest that these therapies do benefit some patients. But not all. Even when there's success, there appears to be a need for constant readjustment, because the pain often returns.

I believe that the inconsistency of chiropractic and muscle therapy lies in their failure to address the other cause of chronic pain: the body's overproduction of pain's biochemical mediators. Two of the most powerful mediators of pain and inflammation are two of the bad eicosanoids: PGE_2 and leukotriene B_4. At the same time, good eicosanoids like PGE_1 inhibit the release of non-eicosanoid pain mediators.

You can stop the production of bad eicosanoids—and thus reduce pain—by using anti-inflammatory drugs, which work by knocking out the synthesis of *all* eicosanoids. Aspirin is the most widely used of these drugs. But while aspirin does decrease levels of PGE_2, it has no effect whatsoever on the production of leukotriene B_4. Neither do the more powerful drugs known as nonsteroidal anti-inflammatory drugs (NSAIDs), such as ibuprofen and naproxen.

To knock out leukotriene B_4, you need the real heavy hitters of pain relief: corticosteroids such as cortisone and prednisone. Unfortunately, as we saw earlier, these drugs also depress the immune system by knocking out all eicosanoids, good and bad. So for the chronic-pain patient, long-term use of corticosteroids presents a terrible dilemma—either risk an immune-deficiency condition or suffer continuing pain.

Of course, there's a way around this dilemma: following a Zone-favorable diet. *This should be the baseline nutritional therapy for reducing the need for long-term drug use in the treatment of chronic pain.*

I've worked with a number of chiropractors and muscle therapists who have their patients follow a Zone-favorable diet in addition to skeletal or muscular adjustments. The results: a vastly more consistent relief from chronic pain.

SKIN DISORDERS

With the exception of some lethal forms of skin cancer, most skin diseases are not life threatening. Still, these diseases do have a negative effect on the quality of life, in terms of both sheer appearance and nagging irritation factors—like itching.

The two most common skin diseases are eczema and psoriasis. The underlying cause of both diseases is an overproduction of bad eicosanoids, particularly leukotriene B_4—the same bad eicosanoid that at higher levels causes chronic pain. The usual treatment for these diseases is topical corticosteroids (the only drug that knocks out leukotrienes), but the conditions usually recur. There's evidence that supplementation with activated essential fatty acids brings some relief, but not with any consistency.

I've found that because it reduces the overproduction of bad eicosanoids such as leukotrienes, a Zone-favorable diet can be beneficial to patients with these annoying skin conditions. And there's an additional benefit: the increased circulation of red blood cells in the skin produces a big improvement in skin color.

An interesting sidebar: Retin-A, the only drug ever shown to reduce the appearance of wrinkles, can be considered a nonspecific stimulator of eicosanoids (nonspecific because it stimulates the production of both good and bad eicosanoids). The good eicosanoids generate increased collagen synthesis in the dermis, and the new collagen production removes the wrinkles by filling in the skin depression.

Unfortunately, Retin-A also stimulates the production of bad eicosanoids that generate an inflammatory response, and this inflammation makes the face look like a lobster. So, like aspirin, Retin-A works by modulating eicosanoid levels, but only at a price.

The best way to improve skin condition over the long term is to follow a Zone-favorable diet. In fact, the first sign of essential fatty-acid deficiency is a dramatic deterioration of the skin.

In this chapter I've presented a long list of chronic diseases, in addition to heart disease and cancer, which I believe are strongly linked to an underlying imbalance of eicosanoids. You can alter eicosanoid levels with drugs like aspirin and corticosteroids that knock out eicosanoids, or by direct injection of good eicosanoids, or by supplementation with activated essential fatty acids. Each of these strategies can potentially reduce the symptoms associated with the diseases.

Unfortunately, though, there is currently no consistent long-term drug therapy for any of these conditions that does not have unwelcome side effects. Still, diet alone—even a Zone-favorable diet—is not an alternative to drug therapy, though it can always be a companion. The object of following a Zone-favorable diet is not to eliminate the use of drugs but to reduce the amounts of drugs required to treat the symptoms of the disease. And I must add this caution: if you're currently taking any medication, never change your diet for better or worse without first contacting your physician. Any dietary change (for better or worse) will affect eicosanoids, and that in turn could possibly affect the amount of medication required to stay within a therapeutic zone.

In some patients, especially those with immunological disturbances, a Zone-favorable diet alone may not be enough. These patients may initially need small amounts of activated essential fatty acids to ensure that adequate levels of these vital substances will be available for eicosanoid formation.

How much is a small amount? It depends on the disease. Cardiovascular conditions, for example, require very little additional activated essential fatty-acid supplementation to a Zone-favorable diet. Autoimmune diseases and fatigue-related conditions require more. In my experience, the baseline for a patient following a Zone-favorable diet is between 1 and 10 mg per day of GLA (rarely more), and at least 20 to 50 times that amount (50 to 500 mg per day) of EPA. Actually, my recommended GLA doses are far lower than those routinely sold in health-food stores. But here is a word of caution. Too much supplementation with or consumption of any omega 6 fatty acid can possibly increase arachidonic acid levels, thereby eliminating any benefits of a Zone-favorable diet. The least amount of supplementation is always the best amount when it comes to a Zone-favorable diet.

I reiterate my belief that following a Zone-favorable diet will pay handsome health rewards for anyone who suffers from any of the diseases discussed in this chapter, as well as for victims of heart disease, diabetes, and cancer. And remember: the only "side effects" that come with a Zone-favorable diet are reduced body fat, increased mental energy, and greater physical performance.

There's one chronic disease I've left until last, and that's the disease that strikes everyone. I'm talking about aging. As America continues to get older and grayer, the incidence of all the other chronic diseases—heart disease, diabetes, cancer, arthritis, obesity, and the rest—will continue to increase. The combination of a fatter America with an older America is a sure-fire prescription for health-care disaster, as an increasingly older population tends to use a disproportionate share of the country's health-care resources. Unless we make dramatic change, these demographic facts of life will be the undoing of our health-care system.

The way this country deals with its aging population and the diseases associated with aging will determine the future of health care and health-care reform. Almost all the chronic diseases that are so burdensome—both to the individual victim and to the health-care system as a whole—can be viewed as simply a consequence of eicosanoid imbalances.

Aging itself can't be reversed, but eicosanoid imbalances certainly can. It can be done through diet, and it can be done in a matter of weeks.

So this is my proposal for the ultimate in health-care reform. Instead of demanding more and more high-tech (and high-cost) intervention, why not take the easiest, the least expensive, and the most effective route? The first step for every individual is to take responsibility for his or her own health. The second and final step: follow the road map to the Zone.

CHAPTER SIXTEEN

THE ZONE AND LIFE EXTENSION

The quest for longer life is as old as life itself. From the ancient Greeks to Ponce de León to the many anonymous scientists who populate the world's research laboratories, thousands of people—some honorable, some whose motives have been questionable at best—have searched for a way to keep death at arm's length for as long as possible. And, indeed, the story of industrial civilization is underwritten by the inexorable lengthening of human life expectancy: from the earlier twenties in Roman times, to the mid-thirties at the time of the American Revolution, to forty only a hundred years ago, to an average of almost eighty today.

Can a Zone-favorable diet system help you live longer? I think it can. Most experts believe that there is a fixed limit to how long animals live, whether you're talking about fruit flies or human beings. For humans, the maximum life span is thought to be approximately 115 years, and it's been that way for the last 100,000 years. How can I state that with such precision? The maximum life span for any species can be approximated by the size of the skull to the total body weight. Those sizes for humans have not changed for the past 100,000 years.

But are these limits really fixed? Probably, but it's possible to get closer to that maximum. Scientists have already found a way to dramatically lengthen life span in animals, and all evidence suggests that what can be done for animals can also be done for humans. What is this magical formula? Very simple: eat less food.

In fact, as long as an animal is supplied with all the essential nutrients it needs (including adequate protein and essential fat), caloric intake can be cut by as much as 40 percent. Not only will the animal live longer—sometimes as much as *twice* as long—but it will be healthier, less vulnerable to disease and to the ravages of aging.

Dietary restriction experiments in animals have been going on for at least sixty years, and they almost always work. In fact, cutting calories (but not essential macronutrients) has significantly extended life span in every species it's been tested on—everything from primitive single-cell pond animals to small mammals, such as rats and mice.

Now under way are dietary-restriction experiments involving some of our closest primate relatives: monkeys and chimpanzees. Although it's too soon to tell if feeding them fewer calories is lengthening these animals' lives, early reports indicate that the monkeys have decreased insulin resistance and lowered blood sugar, both signs of good health.

There are a few indications that dietary restriction may extend human life expectancy in the same way that it extends life span in animals. People on the island of Okinawa, for example, are reported to eat 17 to 40 percent fewer calories than their peers in the rest of Japan. Yet Okinawans have only about 60 percent as much heart disease, stroke, and cancer as the Japanese. And Okinawa is among the world's leading producer of centenarians—people who live one hundred years or more.

There's more evidence. In the 1960s, a team of scientists in Spain reported an experiment with two groups of elderly people in a nursing home. One group ate "normally," while a second group ate a calorie-restricted diet. Over the course of three years, the calorie-restricted group had only half the rate of illness and *half the death rate* of the group who ate their fill.

These scattered reports are indications that dietary restriction may well extend life expectancy in humans. Until now it has been virtually impossible to design an experiment long enough and with enough controls to answer the question scientifically. It's been assumed that it would be very difficult to find people willing to cut their food consumption by 40 percent—that's right on the borderline of starvation—even for a few weeks, let alone for their entire lives.

But the famous (or notorious, depending on your point of view) Biosphere experiment included a living trial of dietary restriction in humans. The Biosphere experiment involved eight people living in a totally enclosed environment for a one-year period. (One of the Biospherians was Dr. Roy Walford, a respected UCLA researcher who has been a leading authority in dietary-restriction studies, and who practices dietary restriction himself.) During the six-month study period, the four men and four women in the Biosphere restricted their intake of calories by 29 percent. During that time, they all registered decreased changes in blood pressure, cholesterol, and triglycerides— changes that were similar to those seen in animal studies. (In fact, the changes were also similar to those our Type II diabetic patients experienced when they followed a Zone-favorable diet. The major difference was that our patients didn't have to live in the Biosphere.)

Even so, the scientists who've been conducting dietary restriction experiments have been thinking calorically, not hormonally. Actually, it should be fairly easy to do a controlled life-extension experiment in humans—as long as you use a Zone-favorable diet. Once a person reaches the Zone, he or she doesn't need as many calories to stay there. (That's because the Zone-favorable diet is helping them access their stored body fat with increasing efficiency.) Once a person reaches his or her ideal percentage of body fat, then they simply start adding enough extra monounsaturated fat to their current Zone-favorable diet to maintain that desired percentage of body fat. On a Zone-favorable diet, caloric intake has basically been reduced to the same levels of total calories needed for humans to follow classic dietary-restriction experiments. For the average person, that will be 800 to 1,200 calories a day. This may seem like a starvation diet, but I guarantee you that you'll have trouble eating all the food necessary to get to those calorie levels if you follow the rules for a Zone-favorable diet.

Of course, you don't have to wait a lifetime to gain the benefits of a Zone-favorable diet. Within two weeks you'll have less hunger, freedom from carbohydrate cravings, greater mental focus, and greater physical performance. A Zone-favorable diet is not a starvation diet; it's a hormonally correct diet.

Let's look at the dietary-restriction experiments, and see what specific effects underfeeding (but not malnutrition) has on these animals' bodies. Once we understand those effects, it's easy to see the implications for humans.

Part of the success of caloric restriction stems from the fact that it takes a lot of energy to digest food and store excess calories, and the process itself creates free radicals. Reducing the number of free radicals reduces the rate of oxidation in the animals' cells, and thus slows down the process of aging.

As I mentioned earlier, the most likely target of excessive levels of free radicals is the essential fatty acids that are the parents of eicosanoids. If you cut down the number of free radicals—something that's automatic with a Zone-favorable diet—you'll see less disturbance of eicosanoid balance.

There are other life-extension benefits that come from reducing the total amount of carbohydrates in the diet. Lower amounts of carbohydrates mean a decreased production of AGEs (advanced glycosylation endproducts), "garbage" substances produced when excess carbohydrate chemically crosslinks with proteins. These AGE products are like a biological form of Krazy Glue—they stick to places they're not supposed to (like arteries and cellular DNA), disrupting their function and thereby accelerating various disease processes.

In humans, the best indicator of the presence of AGE products is glycosylated hemoglobin. You may remember that, in our studies with Type II diabetics, four months of following a Zone-favorable diet reduced levels of this particular AGE product by some 20 percent.

Even more important, reducing calories and carbohydrates will decrease insulin production and the corresponding overproduction of bad eicosanoids. I believe that this is the real key to the superior health and longevity found in animals undergoing calorie restriction.

Same thing in humans. My studies with Type II diabetic patients have shown that insulin levels are reduced by 30 percent after the patients have followed a Zone-favorable diet for four months—the same results you'd expect from an anti-aging diet based on 30 years of research.

That's not all. Remember that with lower levels of insulin the size and mass of fat cells actually shrinks. On consistent calorie-restricted diets, there are no fat rats. On a consistent Zone-favorable diet, there are no fat humans. Ultimately, that means longer life for the heart.

The heart gets other rewards as well. You'll recall that the health of the heart depends on factors like blood pressure and blood flow, and these are ultimately controlled by the balance of good and bad eicosanoids. Calorie restriction reduces blood pressure, which diminishes the risk of heart attacks and strokes. This is exactly what happens when you reach the Zone and stay there over time.

Meanwhile, long-term underfeeding significantly lowers blood levels of cholesterol and triglycerides, which reduces the risk of atherosclerosis and keeps the heart's vital plumbing open and healthy. Again, that's the same result we got when we put Type II diabetics on a Zone-favorable diet.

All this leads me to believe that for humans a Zone-favorable diet should also be viewed as an anti-aging diet that can be easily followed. By this I mean that what other scientists are observing with dietary restriction in animals (and limited human studies) are the same results I've consistently seen with a Zone-favorable diet. The clues are all there: better cardiovascular health, better immune function, better control of insulin—all consequences of better eicosanoid control.

Underlying all this is an inescapable conclusion. Dietary restriction may actually be helping the body to produce more good eicosanoids than bad ones—the same fundamental effect that you'll get from a Zone-favorable diet. In fact, as I've said, the Zone-favorable diet *is* a calorie-restricted diet. But instead of setting a mathematical limit on calories—a limit that doesn't work for real people—a Zone-favorable diet simply puts calorie restriction on automatic pilot. In other words, because the Zone-favorable diet controls insulin, glucagon, and eicosanoids, you simply won't need to eat as much.

With a Zone-favorable diet, you'll still get all the essential nutrients you need (much as in the dietary-restriction experiments), with adequate protein and low levels of fat. But you'll get much more hormonal bang from your calorie buck. So you'll get all the health benefits of dietary restriction without near-starvation—without even having to sacrifice many of your favorite foods. In the short term your quality of life will be significantly improved. In the long term, you might just live long enough to take your great-grandchildren to their first ball game, or hold their hands on the first day of kindergarten.

Great, you say—who wouldn't want to live longer, as long as the extra years are healthy and active? But think about this: you can live a longer life even *without* adding extra years. Nearly one-third of your life is spent in nonfunctional time—sleep. You need to sleep in order to repair and renew your body for the next day. But what if you could speed up that nightly repair process? What would be the immediate effects of simply sleeping less, yet waking up with renewed energy?

If you've already reached the age of forty, it's quite likely that you'll live to be eighty. Let's say you could sleep one hour less each night for the next forty years, thereby giving you an extra hour of functional life each day. That means you'd gain fifteen extra days of functional life each year. Multiply that increase each year by forty years, and you gain 1.7 years of functional life. (If medical science could eliminate all forms of cancer, the result would be about the same increase in life expectancy.) Furthermore, you get your increased life when you want it the most—right now.

Why do I mention this? Because another benefit of being in the Zone is that your needs for sleep will decrease by one to two hours per day. Immediate life extension the easy way.

Of course, long life without good health is not a blessing but a burden. The key is maintaining good health and maximum vitality even in old age. Dietary restriction does that in lab animals. Despite the fact that they live longer, the animals are actually less susceptible to disease than their eat-all-you-want relatives. I think that if you follow the nutritional prescriptions I give you, you'll get exactly the same benefits—long life, increased vitality, and the greatest gift of all: good health.

It's all possible in the Zone.

CHAPTER SEVENTEEN

SUMMING UP

This book represents my personal quest to understand what I can do to prevent my own potential untimely death from heart disease. As long ago as 1982 I knew that the ultimate solution would be a matter of learning how to control eicosanoids and thus control my genetic fate. But how? During the course of my personal odyssey into understanding the nutritional code of eicosanoids, I kept coming back to fundamental common sense—everything in moderation.

The starting point for the development of a Zone-favorable diet was to control eicosanoid balance by fusing drug-delivery technology with sound nutrition principles. But there are other lines of scientific evidence that support the fundamental benefits of a Zone-favorable diet. These points are summarized in Figure 17-1.

First, a Zone-favorable diet is based on humanity's genetic

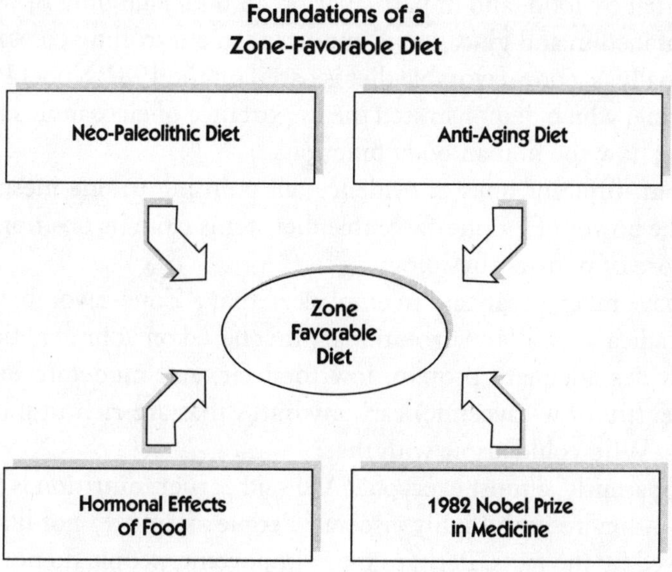

Foundations of a
Zone-Favorable Diet

Neo-Paleolithic Diet

Anti-Aging Diet

Zone
Favorable
Diet

Hormonal Effects
of Food

1982 Nobel Prize
in Medicine

Figure 17-1

makeup. Your genes favor a diet with a relatively constant protein-to-carbohydrate ratio and with most of the carbohydrates being low-density and low-glycemic carbohydrates. In other words, human beings are "designed" by evolution to eat a Zone-favorable diet. Over the past 100,000 years these genes have not changed. A small portion of the population has a genetic capacity to have a blunted insulin response to carbohydrates. Genetically, they're lucky. But most people are simply not designed to eat pasta.

Second, the best way to retard aging is to restrict calories, but not essential nutrients. A Zone-favorable diet is a low-calorie diet that supplies adequate amounts of protein, essential fat, and micronutrients—all crucial for maintaining a high nutritional status. The only two restrictions in a Zone-favorable diet are (1) high-density, high-glycemic carbohydrates like grains, breads, pasta, rice, and other starches; and (2) protein sources rich in arachidonic acid—egg yolks, fatty red meat, and organ meats. (Actually, none of these foods are absolutely forbidden—just use them in moderation. But if you have a disease condition that's linked to eicosanoid disturbances—heart disease, diabetes, cancer, etc.—then you should reduce your consumption of these foods to minimal levels.)

Third, a Zone-favorable diet is based on the hormonal responses generated by food, and in particular on an understanding of why the ratio of insulin and glucagon is important in controlling eicosanoids.

Finally, a Zone-favorable diet is based on the 1982 Nobel Prize in Medicine, which demonstrated the importance of eicosanoids in controlling how the human body functions.

Four different lines of evidence, all pointing to one inescapable fact: the power of a Zone-favorable diet stems from its position at the very core of human physiology.

I have taken great care to emphasize that a Zone-favorable diet is not a radical diet, it's an evolutionary diet based on your genetic code. It provides adequate protein, low total fat, and moderate levels of low-density (low-glycemic) carbohydrates that are rich in micronutrients. Who could argue with that?

Apparently, almost everyone. As I said earlier, nutrition is like religion—they're both highly visceral. People simply do not like to be confused by the facts. Perhaps more important, people do not like to be confronted with concepts that appear alien. Eicosanoids is one such concept—I admit, the word even has an alien sound.

The Zone is not really a diet book, but rather a testimony to the power of food in controlling hormonal response. In this sense, the Zone is not about nutrition, but about twenty-first-century biotechnology. I have purposely tried to walk a fine line between giving detailed scientific descriptions and trying to make this book accessible to the widest possible audience. I've done this because I believe that understanding the implications of the Zone goes to the very heart of what almost everyone wants: to maximize the quality of life.

At the same time, *The Zone* is a wake-up call to all Americans: the dietary recommendations from well-meaning nutrition experts and the government have extremely serious health consequences, especially for people who are genetically unable to handle high-density (high-glycemic) carbohydrates such as pasta and bread. These items simply didn't exist 100,000 years ago.

Unfortunately, these high-density carbohydrates are the foundation of the new dietary guidelines being advocated by nutritional experts and by the government. But the epidemic rise of obesity in this country makes me certain that without a significant change in the public's current overconsumption of high-density carbohydrates, the incidence of heart disease, cancer, and diabetes will begin to skyrocket in the early part of the twenty-first century. I hope that I'm wrong, but I don't think so.

If disease rates do skyrocket, how will we deal with it as a society, as a nation? Presently, our reaction seems to be to reform our health-care system so that everyone who's sick will be guaranteed treatment. But in the final analysis, health-care reform has nothing to do with increasing the availability of MRI scans or obtaining cheaper health insurance. True health-care reform begins when an individual finally begins to take responsibility for his or her own health, and stops abdicating that responsibility to a third party—whether it be the government, an insurance company, or even a personal physician. I hope this book provides a state-of-the-art, user-friendly how-to guide to reach that goal.

I fully expect that all the key facts presented in this book will become lightning rods for controversy, if only because they've not been thoroughly understood. So let me repeat them:

- *Despite eating less fat, Americans are fatter than ever.* Why? Because fat does not make you fat, insulin does. There are two ways to increase insulin—eat too much food at any one meal, or eat too many carbohydrates. Americans do both simultaneously.

• *Eating fat doesn't make you fat, as long as it's the right type of fat.* Monounsaturated fat has no effect on insulin. On the other hand, saturated fat can increase insulin by causing the condition known as insulin resistance.

A Zone-favorable diet is rich in monounsaturated fat, and is designed to generate the production of good eicosanoids, both of which will moderate insulin levels. However, if you're eating too many carbohydrates, adding *any* type of fat is a real prescription for rapid fat gain.

• *Athletes perform better on a high-fat diet than on a high-carbohydrate diet.* Eating a high-carbohydrate diet is a guarantee that athletes will never reach their full genetic performance potential. The hormonal consequences of elevated insulin and the resulting overproduction of bad eicosanoids impact negatively on athletic performance and training.

• *Exercise alone will rarely overcome the negative effects of a high-carbohydrate diet.* The food you eat is your main ticket to get and stay in the Zone. This is not to to say don't exercise. Exercise is a great hormonal modulator, and it can help keep you in the Zone, but it takes a lot of exercise to undo the negative hormonal effects of a high-carbohydrate diet. What's the best form of exercise? Anything you do on a consistent basis. For most people, that will be walking.

• *For cardiovascular patients, a high-carbohydrate diet may be hazardous to their health.* Almost by definition, cardiovascular patients suffer from elevated insulin levels. A high-carbohydrate diet, especially for those patients with a genetically elevated insulin response to carbohydrates, can only increase insulin levels, and *elevated insulin is the greatest predictor of the likelihood of a heart attack.*

• *Food may be the most powerful drug you will ever take.* Hormones are hundreds of times stronger than drugs. Every time you eat, you start a hormonal cascade. Either you control it, or for the next four to six hours it controls you.

• *The new dietary recommendations of the U.S. government, nutrition experts, and medical experts are dead wrong.* The new food pyramid, which has as its base high-density carbohydrates, will for many people be a prescription for elevated insulin (hyperinsulinemia)—thus moving them further and further away from the Zone. If the base of the new food pyramid were simply thrown away, you'd be left with a Zone-favorable diet.

• *The quality of your life is controlled by the Zone.* Less excess body fat, greater mental productivity, better physical performance, and a decreased likelihood of chronic diseases are the essence of a better quality of life. These are also the results of being in the Zone. If you're willing to treat food with the same precision as you would a drug prescription, then your access to the Zone is guaranteed. In the Zone, you can modify the expression of your genetic destiny, ultimately reaching your full genetic potential.

Don't be misled by the apparent simplicity of this dietary program to reach the Zone. A Zone-favorable diet, if properly followed, produces fundamental changes at the hormonal level that everyone can achieve. This program is designed to orchestrate a vast array of powerful hormonal responses, responses that have evolved over the past forty million years. Many of the ancient strategies (diet, exercise, stress reduction, etc.) that have filtered down into modern medicine can now be explained by understanding how they operate at the hormonal level in general, and in particular by how they affect eicosanoids. You have to eat. You might as well eat a diet that's hormonally correct.

Of course, people often will not change their diet patterns even if they know that change will improve their quality of life. Why? They don't want to stop eating the foods they like. It's too hard to remember what to eat and what not to eat. And they're totally confused by conflicting advice about nutrition.

I've been aware of these problems for a long time, and I think I've developed solutions for all of them, solutions that are presented throughout this book.

Problem one: you can still eat the foods you like on a Zone-favorable diet. Just follow my macronutrient block program, at the same time maintaining the appropriate balance of protein to carbohydrate. You just have to pay a little more attention to the amounts of protein and carbohydrate you eat at each meal.

Problem two: there's not much to remember on a Zone-favorable diet. All you have to remember is the block sizes of the foods you like to eat. It's probably harder to remember your telephone number.

Problem three: current nutritional research is like twelve blind-folded people trying to describe an elephant—each person touches one part, and tries to explain the whole elephant in terms of that part. Once you've mastered the language of eicosanoids, it's as if all the blindfolds have been taken off—your confusion about nutrition will simply evaporate.

An understanding of how eicosanoids are controlled by diet will be the foundation of the next frontier in twenty-first-century medicine. Eventually, as more and more physicians learn this basic concept (and hope I this book will start them in that direction), I believe that the hormonal benefits gained from a Zone-favorable diet will be considered the primary treatment for all chronic disease states, with drugs being used as secondary backup.

In other words, *once the medical establishment finally understands the potential of diet to alter eicosanoids, that should revolutionize the current practice of medicine.*

Obviously, this won't happen overnight. It will require a substantial educational effort to develop a common language based on eicosanoids, and at the moment that language is all but unknown. But once developed, it will eventually tie together observations from the earliest days of recorded history with the most recent advances in medicine. Without that common language, we have a medical Tower of Babel. The resulting confusion prevents a consistent, total approach to optimal health.

At the core of the Zone are some very complex biochemical concepts. Yet the power of the Zone is that anyone can begin to tap into this hormonal control technology simply by following the dietary steps outlined in this book. But this requires that you take charge of your life. You have to make the time to keep your body in the Zone. If you don't, then you'll never reach wellness, let alone optimum health.

Optimal health means maximizing the quality of your life. Your goal may not be to reach the maximum human life span of 115 years, but to squeeze every bit out of life within your allotted time on this planet.

I've tried to give you some of the rules and some of the tools I have developed to plot your own course to the Zone. But only you can actually start to use them. As I tell everyone, I don't care if it's a drug, a diet, a vitamin, or a mineral. If you try any new program for two weeks, and you don't see a significant difference in how you feel, then it probably isn't going to happen. Following a Zone-favorable diet is no different. All you have to give it is two weeks of your time.

As the president of a successful biotechnology company, I'm putting my scientific reputation on the line every time someone follows this dietary program.

Since it's my reputation, I'll make you an offer: if you have any problems following the guidelines in this book, simply call me at my toll-free number listed in Appendix A and my staff will work with you. Likewise, if you're a physician and want more information on eicosanoids, give me a call. I'll be more than glad to help you understand them. Through my own understanding of eicosanoids I now hold my own genetic destiny in my hands.

I hope you will too.

TECHNICAL SUPPORT

My scientific reputation is on the line when you follow a Zone-favorable diet as I have outlined. If you would like additional information, have any questions, or have any initial difficulties with a Zone-favorable diet, call 1-800-346-2703 and a member of my staff will work with you. If you're a physician and desire additional medical information, simply call 1-800-346-2703 and a member of my staff will handle your requests.

I can also be directly contacted by mail addressed to Dr. Barry Sears, Eicotech Corporation at 21 Tioga Way, Marblehead, MA 01945.

CALCULATION OF LEAN BODY MASS

A rapid way to determine your lean body mass is simply to use a tape measure and scale. You should make all measurements on bare skin (not through clothing), and make sure that the tape fits snugly but does not compress the skin and underlying tissue. Take all measurements three times and calculate the average. All measurements should be in inches. The tables used to calculate the percentage of body fat were used with the permission of Dr. Michael Eades from his book *Thin So Fast*.

CALCULATING BODY-FAT PERCENTAGES FOR FEMALES

There are five steps you must take to calculate your percentage of body fat:

1. While keeping the tape level, measure your hips at their widest point, and your waist at the umbilicus (i.e., belly button). It is critical that you measure at the belly button and not at the narrowest point of your waist. Take each of these measurements three times and compute the average.
2. Measure your height in inches without shoes.
3. Record your height, waist, and hip measurements on the accompanying worksheet.
4. Find each of these measurements in the appropriate column in the accompanying tables and record the constants on the worksheet.
5. Add constants A and B, then subtract constant C for this sum and round to the nearest whole number. That figure is your percentage of body fat.

WORKSHEET FOR WOMEN TO CALCULATE THEIR PERCENTAGE OF BODY FAT

Average hip measurement _____ (used for Constant A)

Average abdomen measurement _____ (used for Constant B)

Height _____ (used for Constant C)

Using Table 1, look up each of the average measurements and your height in the appropriate column.

Constant A = _____

Constant B = _____

Constant C = _____

To determine your approximate percentage of body fat, then add Constant A and B. From that total, subtract Constant C. The result is your percentage of body fat.

CALCULATING BODY-FAT PERCENTAGES FOR MEN

There are four steps you must take to determine your body-fat percentage:

1. While keeping the tape level, measure the circumference of your waist at the umbilicus (i.e., belly button). Measure three times and compute the average.
2. Measure your wrist at the space between your dominant hand and your wrist bone, at the location where your wrist bends.
3. Record these measurements on the worksheet for males.
4. Subtract your wrist measurement from your waist measurement and find the resulting value listed in the table. On the left-hand side of this table, find your weight. Proceed to right

from your weight and down from your waist-minus-wrist measurement. Where these two points intersect, read your body fat percentage.

WORKSHEET FOR MEN TO CALCULATE THEIR PERCENTAGE OF BODY FAT

Average waist measurement   _____   (inches)

Average wrist measurement   _____   (inches)

Subtract the wrist measurement from the waist measurement. Use Table 2 to find your weight. Then find your "waist minus wrist" number. Where the two columns intersect is your approximate percentage of body fat.

CALCULATING LEAN BODY MASS FOR BOTH FEMALES AND MALES

Now that you know your body-fat percentage, the next step is to use this figure to calculate the weight in pounds of the fat portion of your total body weight. This is done by multiplying your weight by your percentage of body fat (Remember to use a decimal point—15 percent is 0.15 for example).

(Weight) × (% of body fat) = total body-fat weight

Once you know the weight of your total body fat, you subtract that total fat weight from your total weight, which results in your lean body mass. Lean body mass is the total weight of all nonfat body tissue.

_____Your total weight
- _____Your total of body fat
= _____Your lean body mass

Lean body mass = total weight – total body-fat weight

TABLE 1

Conversion Constants for Prediction of Percentage of Body Fat in Females

HIPS		ABDOMEN		HEIGHT	
INCHES	CONSTANT A	INCHES	CONSTANT B	INCHES	CONSTANT C
30	33.48	20	14.22	55	33.52
30.5	33.83	20.5	14.40	55.5	33.67
31	34.87	21.0	14.93	56	34.13
31.5	35.22	21.5	15.11	56.5	34.28
32	36.27	22	15.64	57	34.74
32.5	36.62	22.5	15.82	57.5	34.89
33	37.67	23	16.35	58	35.35
33.5	38.02	23.5	16.53	58.5	35.50
34	39.06	24	17.06	59	35.96
34.5	39.41	24.5	17.24	59.5	36.11
35	40.46	25	17.78	60	36.57
35.5	40.81	25.5	17.96	60.5	36.72
36	41.86	26	18.49	61	37.18
36.5	42.21	26.5	18.67	61.5	37.33
37	43.25	27	19.20	62	37.79
37.5	43.60	27.5	19.38	62.5	37.94
38	44.65	28	19.91	63	38.40
38.5	45.32	28.5	20.27	63.5	38.70
39	46.05	29	20.62	64	39.01
39.5	46.40	29.5	20.80	64.5	39.16
40	47.44	30	21.33	65	39.62
40.5	47.79	30.5	21.51	65.5	39.77
41	48.84	31	22.04	66	40.23
41.5	49.19	31.5	22.22	66.5	40.38
42	50.24	32	22.75	67	40.84
42.5	50.59	32.5	22.93	67.5	40.99
43	51.64	33	23.46	68	41.45
43.5	51.99	33.5	23.64	68.5	41.60
44	53.03	34	24.18	69	42.06
44.5	53.41	34.5	24.36	69.5	42.21

HIPS		ABDOMEN		HEIGHT	
INCHES	CONSTANT A	INCHES	CONSTANT B	INCHES	CONSTANT C
45	54.53	35	24.89	70	42.67
45.5	54.86	35.5	25.07	70.5	42.82
46	55.83	36	25.60	71	43.28
46.5	56.18	36.5	25.78	71.5	43.43
47	57.22	37	26.31	72	43.89
47.5	57.57	37.5	26.49	72.5	44.04
48	58.62	38	27.02	73	44.50
48.5	58.97	38.5	27.20	73.5	44.65
49	60.02	39	27.73	74	45.11
49.5	60.37	39.5	27.91	74.5	45.26
50	61.42	40	28.44	75	45.72
50.5	61.77	40.5	28.62	75.5	45.87
51	62.81	41	29.15	76	46.32
51.5	63.16	41.5	29.33		
52	64.21	42	29.87		
52.5	64.56	42.5	30.05		
53	65.61	43	30.58		
53.5	65.96	43.5	30.76		
54	67.00	44	31.29		
54.5	67.35	44.5	31.47		
55	68.40	45	32.00		
55.5	68.75	45.5	32.18		
56	69.80	46	32.71		
56.5	70.15	46.5	32.89		
57	71.19	47	33.42		
57.5	71.54	47.5	33.60		
58	72.59	48	34.13		
58.5	72.94	48.5	34.31		
59	73.99	49	34.84		
59.5	74.34	49.5	35.02		
60	75.39	50	35.56		

TABLE 2

Male Percentage Body Fat Calculations

Waist-Wrist (in inches)	22	22.5	23	23.5	24
Weight (in lbs.)					
120	4	6	8	10	12
125	4	6	7	9	11
130	3	5	7	9	11
135	3	5	7	8	10
140	3	5	6	8	10
145		4	6	7	9
150		4	6	7	9
155		4	5	6	8
160		4	5	6	8
165		3	5	6	8
170		3	4	6	7
175			4	6	7
180			4	5	7
185			4	5	6
190			4	5	6
195			3	5	6
200			3	4	6
205				4	5
210				4	5
215				4	5
220				4	5
225				3	4
230				3	4
235				3	4
240					4
245					4
250					4
255					3
260					3
265					
270					
275					
280					
285					
290					
295					
300					

24.5	25	25.5	26	26.5	27	27.5
14	16	18	20	21	23	25
13	15	17	19	20	22	24
12	14	16	18	20	21	23
12	13	15	17	19	20	22
11	13	15	16	18	19	21
11	12	14	15	17	19	20
10	12	13	15	16	18	19
10	11	13	14	16	17	19
9	11	12	14	15	17	18
9	10	12	13	15	16	17
9	10	11	13	14	15	17
8	10	11	12	12	15	16
8	9	10	12	13	14	16
8	9	10	11	13	14	15
7	8	10	11	12	13	15
7	8	9	11	12	13	14
7	8	9	10	11	12	14
6	8	9	10	11	12	13
6	7	8	9	11	12	13
6	7	8	9	10	11	12
6	7	8	9	10	11	12
6	7	8	9	10	11	12
5	6	7	8	9	10	11
5	6	7	8	9	10	11
5	6	7	8	9	10	11
5	6	7	8	9	9	10
5	6	6	7	8	9	10
4	5	6	7	8	9	10
4	5	6	7	8	9	10
4	5	6	7	8	8	9
4	5	6	7	7	8	9
4	5	5	6	7	8	9
4	4	5	6	7	8	9
4	4	5	6	7	8	8
3	4	5	6	7	7	8
3	4	5	6	6	7	8
3	4	5	5	6	7	8

Waist-Wrist (in inches)	28	28.5	29	29.5	30	30.5	31
Weight (in lbs.)							
120	27	29	31	33	35	37	39
125	26	28	30	32	33	35	37
130	25	27	28	30	32	34	36
135	24	26	27	29	31	32	34
140	23	24	26	28	29	31	33
145	22	23	25	27	28	30	31
150	21	23	24	26	27	29	30
155	20	22	23	25	26	28	29
160	19	21	22	24	25	27	28
165	19	20	22	23	24	26	27
170	18	19	21	22	24	25	26
175	17	19	20	21	23	24	25
180	17	18	19	21	22	23	25
185	16	18	19	20	21	23	24
190	16	17	18	19	21	22	23
195	15	16	18	19	20	21	22
200	15	16	17	18	19	21	22
205	14	15	17	18	19	20	21
210	14	15	16	17	18	19	21
215	13	15	16	17	18	19	20
220	13	14	15	16	17	18	19
225	13	14	15	16	17	18	19
230	12	13	14	15	16	17	18
235	12	13	14	15	16	17	18
240	12	13	14	15	16	17	17
245	11	12	13	14	15	16	17
250	11	12	13	14	15	16	17
255	11	12	13	14	14	15	16
260	10	11	12	13	14	15	16
265	10	11	12	13	14	15	15
270	10	11	12	13	13	14	15
275	10	11	11	12	13	14	15
280	9	10	11	12	13	14	14
285	9	10	11	12	12	13	14
290	9	10	11	11	12	13	14
295	9	10	10	11	12	13	14
300	9	9	10	11	12	12	13

31.5	32	32.5	33	33.5	34	34.5
41	43	45	47	49	50	52
39	41	43	45	46	48	50
37	39	41	43	44	46	48
36	38	39	41	43	44	46
34	36	38	39	41	43	44
33	35	36	38	39	41	43
32	33	35	36	38	40	41
31	32	34	35	37	38	40
30	31	33	34	35	37	38
29	30	31	33	34	36	37
28	29	30	32	33	34	36
27	28	29	31	32	33	35
26	27	28	30	31	32	34
25	26	28	29	30	31	33
24	26	27	28	29	30	32
24	25	26	27	28	30	31
23	24	25	26	28	29	30
22	23	25	26	27	28	29
22	23	24	25	26	27	28
21	22	23	24	25	26	28
20	22	23	24	25	26	27
20	21	22	23	24	25	26
19	20	21	22	23	24	25
19	20	21	22	23	24	25
18	19	20	21	22	23	24
18	19	20	21	22	23	24
18	18	19	20	21	22	23
17	18	19	20	21	22	23
17	18	19	19	20	21	22
16	17	18	19	20	21	22
16	17	18	19	19	20	21
16	16	17	18	19	20	21
15	16	17	18	19	19	20
15	16	17	17	18	19	20
15	15	16	17	18	19	19
14	15	16	17	17	18	19
14	15	16	16	17	18	19

Waist-Wrist (in inches)	35	35.5	36	36.5	37
Weight (in lbs.)					
120	54				
125	52	54			
130	50	52	53	55	
135	48	50	51	53	55
140	46	48	49	51	53
145	44	46	47	49	51
150	43	44	46	47	49
155	41	43	44	46	47
160	40	41	43	44	46
165	38	40	41	43	44
170	37	39	40	41	43
175	36	37	39	40	41
180	35	36	37	39	40
185	34	35	36	38	39
190	33	34	35	37	38
195	32	33	34	35	37
200	31	32	33	35	36
205	30	31	32	34	35
210	29	30	32	33	34
215	29	30	31	32	33
220	28	29	30	31	32
225	27	28	29	30	31
230	26	27	28	30	31
235	26	27	28	29	30
240	25	26	27	28	29
245	25	26	27	27	28
250	24	25	26	27	28
255	24	24	25	26	27
260	23	24	25	26	27
265	22	23	24	25	26
270	22	23	24	25	25
275	22	22	23	24	25
280	21	22	23	24	24
285	21	21	22	23	24
290	20	21	22	23	23
295	20	21	21	22	23
300	19	20	21	22	22

37.5	38	38.5	39	39.5	40	40.5
54						
52	54	55				
50	52	53	55			
49	50	52	53	55		
47	48	50	51	53	54	
45	47	48	50	51	52	54
44	45	47	48	49	51	52
43	44	45	47	48	49	51
41	43	44	45	47	48	49
40	41	43	44	45	46	48
39	40	41	43	44	45	46
38	39	40	41	43	44	45
37	38	39	40	41	43	44
36	37	38	39	40	41	43
35	36	37	38	39	40	42
34	35	36	37	38	39	40
33	34	35	36	37	38	39
32	33	34	35	36	37	38
32	33	34	35	36	37	38
31	32	33	34	35	36	37
30	31	32	33	34	35	36
29	30	31	32	33	34	35
29	30	31	31	32	33	34
28	29	30	31	32	33	34
27	28	29	30	31	32	33
27	28	29	29	30	31	32
26	27	28	29	30	31	31
26	27	27	28	29	30	31
25	26	27	28	29	29	30
25	26	26	27	28	29	30
24	25	26	27	27	28	29
24	25	25	26	27	28	28
23	24	25	26	26	27	28

Waist-Wrist (in inches)	41	41.5	42	42.5	43	43.5
Weight (in lbs.)						
120						
125						
130						
135						
140						
145						
150						
155						
160						
165	55					
170	54	55				
175	52	53	55			
180	50	52	53	54		
185	49	50	51	53	54	55
190	48	49	50	51	52	54
195	46	47	49	50	51	52
200	45	46	47	48	50	51
205	44	45	46	47	48	49
210	43	44	45	46	47	48
215	42	43	44	45	46	47
220	41	42	43	44	45	46
225	40	41	42	43	44	45
230	39	40	41	42	44	44
235	38	39	40	41	42	43
240	37	38	39	40	41	42
245	36	37	38	39	40	41
250	35	36	37	38	39	40
255	34	35	36	37	38	39
260	34	35	35	36	37	38
265	33	34	35	36	36	37
270	32	33	34	35	36	37
275	32	32	33	34	35	36
280	31	32	33	33	34	35
285	30	31	32	33	34	34
290	30	31	31	32	33	34
295	29	30	31	32	32	33
300	29	29	30	31	32	33

44	44.5	45	45.5	46	46.5	47
55						
53	55					
52	53	54	55			
51	52	53	54	55		
49	50	51	53	54	55	
48	49	50	51	52	53	54
47	48	49	50	51	52	53
46	47	48	49	50	51	52
45	46	47	48	49	50	51
44	45	46	47	48	49	50
43	44	45	46	46	47	48
42	43	44	44	45	46	47
41	42	43	44	44	45	46
40	41	42	43	44	44	45
39	40	41	42	43	43	44
38	39	40	41	42	43	43
37	38	39	40	41	42	43
37	38	38	39	40	41	42
36	37	38	38	39	40	41
35	36	37	38	39	39	40
35	35	36	37	38	39	39
34	35	36	36	37	38	39
33	34	35	36	36	37	38

Waist-Wrist (in inches)	47.5	48	48.5	49	49.5	50
Weight (in lbs.)						
120						
125						
130						
135						
140						
145						
150						
155						
160						
165						
170						
175						
180						
185						
190						
195						
200						
205						
210						
215	55					
220	54	55				
225	53	54	55			
230	52	53	54	55		
235	51	51	52	53	54	55
240	49	50	51	52	53	54
245	48	49	50	51	52	53
250	47	48	49	50	51	52
255	46	47	48	49	50	51
260	45	46	47	48	49	50
265	44	45	46	47	48	49
270	43	44	45	46	47	48
275	43	43	44	45	46	47
280	42	43	43	44	45	46
285	41	42	43	43	44	45
290	40	41	42	43	43	44
295	39	40	41	42	43	43
300	39	39	40	41	42	43

MACRONUTRIENT FOOD BLOCKS

The concept of macronutrient food blocks gives a straightforward method to construct Zone-favorable meals. Listed below are the sizes of various blocks of protein, carbohydrate, and fat each consisting of one block. The protein blocks are for uncooked portions. Although favorable carbohydrates are usually low-glycemic carbohydrates, there are exceptions (like ice cream and potato chips) which are also high in fat.

I have rounded off the blocks to convenient sizes for easy memory. This list is by no means meant to be exhaustive. If you have a favorite food not listed, refer to Corinne T. Netzer's *Complete Book of Food Counts* (Dell Books) to expand the list.

When constructing a Zone-favorable meal, always remember the primary rule: keep the protein and carbohydrate blocks in a 1:1 ratio.

Protein Blocks (approximately 7 grams protein per block)

MEAT AND POULTRY

Best choice

Chicken breast, deli style	1.5 oz.
Chicken breast, skinless	1 oz.
Turkey breast, deli-style	1.5 oz.
Turkey breast, skinless	1 oz.
Veal	1 oz.

Fair choice

Beef, lean cuts	1 oz.

Canadian bacon, lean	1 oz.
Chicken, dark meat, skinless	1 oz.
Corned beef, lean	1 oz.
Duck	1.5 oz.
Ham, deli style	1.5 oz.
Ham, lean	1 oz.
Lamb, lean	1 oz.
Pork, lean	1 oz.
Pork chop	1 oz.
Turkey, dark meat, skinless	1 oz.
Turkey bacon	3 strips

Poor choice

Bacon	3 strips
Beef, fatty cuts	1 oz.
Beef, ground (more than 10% fat)	1.5 oz.
Hot dog (pork or beef)	1 link
Hot dog (turkey or chicken)	1 link
Kielbasa	2 oz.
Liver, beef	1 oz.
Liver, chicken	1 oz.
Pepperoni	1 oz.
Pork sausage	2 links
Salami	1 oz.

FISH AND SEAFOOD

Bass	1.5 oz.
Bluefish	1.5 oz.
Calamari	2.5 oz.
Catfish	1.5 oz.
Cod	1.5 oz.
Clams	1.5 oz.
Crabmeat	1.5 oz.
Haddock	1.5 oz.
Halibut	1.5 oz.
Lobster	1.5 oz.

Mackerel*	1.5 oz.
Salmon*	1.5 oz.
Sardines*	1 oz.
Scallops	1.5 oz.
Shrimp	1.5 oz.
Snapper	1.5 oz.
Swordfish	1.5 oz.
Trout	1.5 oz.
Tuna (steak)	1.5 oz.
Tuna, canned in water	1 oz.

EGGS

Best choice

Egg whites	2
Egg substitute	¼ cup

Poor choice

Whole egg	1

PROTEIN-RICH DAIRY

Best choice

Cheese, fat free	1 oz.
Cottage cheese, low fat	¼ cup
Cottage cheese, no fat	¼ cup

Fair choice

Cheese, reduced fat	1 oz.
Mozzarella cheese, skim	1 oz.
Ricotta cheese, skim	2 oz.

Poor choice

Hard cheeses	1 oz.

---

*Rich in EPA.

VEGETARIAN

Protein powder	⅓ oz.
Soy burgers	½ patty
Soy hot dog	1 link
Soy sausages	2 links
Tofu, firm or extra firm	1 oz.

MIXED PROTEIN-CARBOHYDRATE (contains one block of protein and one block of carbohydrate)

Milk, low-fat (1%)	1 cup
Tempeh	1.5 oz.
Yogurt, plain	½ cup
Tofu, soft	3 oz.

Carbohydrate Blocks (approximately 9 grams carbohydrate per block)

Favorable Carbohydrates (use primarily)

Cooked vegetables

Artichoke	1 medium
Asparagus	1 cup (12 spears)
Beans, black (canned)	¼ cup
Beans, green or wax	1 cup
Bok choy	3 cups
Broccoli	1 cup
Brussels sprouts	1 cup
Cabbage	1 ½ cups
Cauliflower	2 cups
Chickpeas	¼ cup

Collard greens	1 cup
Eggplant	1½ cups
Kale	1 cup
Kidney beans (canned)	¼ cup
Leeks	1 cup
Lentils	¼ cup
Mushrooms (boiled)	1 cup
Okra, sliced	1 cup
Onions (boiled)	½ cup
Sauerkraut	1 cup
Spinach	1 cup
Swiss chard	1 cup
Turnip, mashed	1 cup
Turnip greens	1½ cups
Yellow squash	1 cup
Zucchini	1 cup

Raw vegetables

Alfalfa sprouts	7½ cups
Bean sprouts	3 cups
Broccoli	2 cups
Cabbage, shredded	2 cups
Cauliflower	2 cups
Celery, sliced	2 cups
Cucumber	1
Cucumber, sliced	3 cups
Endive, chopped	5 cups
Escarole, chopped	5 cups
Green pepper, chopped	1½ cups
Green peppers	2
Hummus	¼ cup
Lettuce, iceberg	1 head

Lettuce, romaine, chopped	6 cups
Mushrooms, chopped	3 cups
Onion, chopped	1 cup
Radishes, sliced	2 cups
Salsa	½ cup
Snow peas	1 cup
Spinach	4 cups
Spinach salad	1

(2 cups raw spinach, ¼ cup raw onion, ¼ cup raw mushrooms, and ¼ cup raw tomato)

Tomato, chopped	1 cup
Tomatoes	2
Tossed salad	1

(2 cups shredded lettuce, ¼ cup raw green pepper, ¼ cup raw cucumber, and ¼ cup raw tomato)

Water chestnuts	½ cup

Fruit (fresh, frozen, or canned light)

Apple	½
Applesauce	¼ cup
Apricots	3
Blackberries	½ cup
Blueberries	½ cup
Cantaloupe	¼ melon
Cantaloupe, cubed	1 cup
Cherries	7
Fruit cocktail	½ cup
Grapefruit	½
Grapes	½ cup
Honeydew melon, cubed	½ cup

Kiwi	1
Lemon	1
Lime	1
Nectarine	½
Orange	½
Orange, mandarin, canned	⅓ cup
Peach	1
Peaches, canned	½ cup
Pear	⅓
Pineapple, cubed	½ cup
Plum	1
Raspberries	⅔ cup
Strawberries	1 cup
Tangerine	1
Watermelon, cubed	½ cup

Grains

Oatmeal, slow cooking*	⅓ cup (cooked) or ½ oz. (dry)

UNFAVORABLE CARBOHYDRATES (use in moderation)

Cooked vegetables

Acorn squash	¼ cup
Baked beans	⅛ cup
Beets, sliced	½ cup
Butternut squash	⅓ cup
Carrots, sliced	½ cup
Corn	¼ cup
Lima beans	¼ cup
Parsnip	⅓ cup

---

*Contains GLA.

Peas	⅓ cup
Pinto beans (canned)	⅓ cup
Potato, baked	⅓ cup
Potato, boiled	⅓ cup
Potato, french fried	5 pieces
Potato, mashed	⅕ cup
Refried beans	¼ cup
Sweet potato, baked	⅓
Sweet potato, mashed	⅕ cup

Fruit

Banana	⅓
Cranberries	¼ cup
Cranberry sauce	4 tsp.
Dates	2
Fig	1
Guava, cubed	½ cup
Kumquat	3
Mango, sliced	⅓ cup
Papaya, cubed	½ cup
Prunes	2
Raisins	1 tbs.

Fruit juices

Apple cider	⅓ cup
Apple juice	¼ cup
Cranberry juice	¼ cup
Fruit punch	¼ cup
Grape juice	½ cup
Grapefruit juice	⅓ cup
Lemon juice	⅓ cup
Lemonade	⅓ cup
Orange juice	⅓ cup

Pineapple juice	¼ cup
Tomato juice	¾ cup
V-8 juice	¾ cup

Grains and Breads

Bagel (small)	¼
Biscuit	¼
Bread, whole-grain	½ slice
Bread, white	½ slice
Bread crumbs	½ oz.
Breadstick	1
Buckwheat, dry	½ oz.
Bulgur wheat, dry	½ oz.
Cereal, dry	½ oz.
Cornbread	1 square
Cornstarch	4 tsp.
Couscous	½ oz.
Croissant, plain	¼
Crouton	½ oz.
Donut, plain	¼
English muffin	¼
Granola	½ oz.
Grits, cooked	⅓ cup
Melba toast	½ oz.
Millet	½ oz.
Muffin, blueberry	¼
Noodles, egg (cooked)	¼ cup
Pancake (4-inch)	½
Pasta, cooked	¼ cup
Pita bread	¼ pocket
Pita bread, mini	½ pocket

Popcorn, popped	2 cups
Rice, brown (cooked)	⅕ cup
Rice, white (cooked)	⅕ cup
Rice cake	1
Roll, dinner	½ small
Roll, hamburger	¼
Taco shell	1
Tortilla, corn (6-inch)	1
Tortilla, flour (8-inch)	½
Waffle	½

Others

Barbecue sauce	2 tbls.
Candy bar	¼
Catsup	2 tbls.
Cocktail sauce	2 tbls.
Cracker (graham)	1
Crackers (saltine)	4
Honey	½ tbls.
Ice cream, premium	⅙ cup
Ice cream, regular	¼ cup
Jam or jelly	2 tsp.
Molasses	2 tsp.
Plum sauce	1½ tbls.
Potato chips	½ oz.
Pretzels	½ oz.
Relish, pickle	4 tsp.
Sugar, brown	1½ tsp.
Sugar, confectioners'	1 tbls.

Sugar,	
granulated	2 tsp.
Syrup, maple	2 tsp.
Syrup, pancake	2 tsp.
Teriyaki sauce	½ oz.
Tortilla chips	½ oz.

FAT

Best choice (rich in monounsaturated fat)

Almond butter	½ tsp.
Almonds (slivered)	1 tsp.
Avocado	½ tbs.
Canola oil	⅓ tsp.
Guacamole	½ tbs.
Macadamia nuts	1
Olive oil	⅓ tsp.
Olive oil and vinegar dressing	1 tsp.
Olives	3
Peanut butter, natural	½ tsp.
Peanut oil	⅓ tsp.
Peanuts	6
Tahini	½ tbls.

Fair choice (low in saturated fat)

Mayonnaise, light	1 tsp.
Mayonnaise, regular	⅓ tsp.
Sesame oil	⅓ tsp.
Soybean oil	⅓ tsp.
Walnuts	½ tsp.

Poor choice (rich in saturated fat)

Bacon bits (imitation)	2 tsp.
Butter	⅓ tsp.
Cream	½ tbls.
Cream cheese	1 tsp.
Cream cheese, light	2 tsp.
Lard	⅓ tsp.
Sour cream	½ tbls.
Sour cream, light	1 tbls.
Vegetable shortening	⅓ tsp.

ZONE-FAVORABLE RECIPES

Gourmet cooking in the Zone is not difficult. With the help of Jeannette Pothier and Ann Rislove, you can prepare some very exciting Zone-favorable meals.

Jeannette is a professional chef with a teaching degree in culinary arts and was associated for ten years with Boston's most renowned chef, Madeleine Kamman, at the Modern Gourmet Cooking School. She was head chef at Café l'Orange in Concord, Massachusetts. Jeannette also trained at the Luberon College in Aix-en-Provence.

Listed below are some of Jeannette's and Ann's favorite recipes.

POACHED HADDOCK WITH HOT GREEN BEANS AND ARTICHOKES
(Serves 4)

Haddock and other similar fish fillets may be baked, broiled, or poached. Poaching is a liquid cooking method, which results in a very moist and delicate piece of fish. The cooking liquid is used to create a simple flavorful white sauce.

1 cup water
½ cup onion, sliced thin
2 cups 2-percent milk
¼ teaspoon sea salt
Pepper
4 haddock fillets, each weighing 4 ounces

Sauce:
1½ tablespoons butter
1½ tablespoons flour
1 cup poaching liquid
20 green grapes, optional

In a large skillet, preferably stainless steel or enameled cast iron, bring the water and onion to a boil. Add the milk, salt, and pepper, and add the fish fillets. Reduce the heat and cook for 5 or 6 minutes. Turn off the heat and remove the fillets to a warm platter.

Over medium heat, reduce the poaching liquid by half. Meanwhile, prepare the sauce. In a small saucepan, over medium heat, melt the butter. Add the flour and cook for a minute, while whisking, to cook the flour. Whisk in half the cup of poaching liquid. The sauce will thicken immediately. Add the rest of the liquid and whisk well. Add green grapes and return the sauce to a boil. Adjust the seasoning and serve the sauce with Hot Green Beans and Artichokes over the fish and garnish with parsley.

HOT GREEN BEANS AND ARTICHOKES
(Serves 4)

Marinade:
3 tablespoons lemon juice
⅓ cup red wine vinegar
¼ cup olive oil
Chopped herbs
Parsley
Chives

18 ounces french green beans
1 cup drained artichoke hearts
1 tablespoon olive oil
½ cup chopped parsley
¼ cup chopped chives
2 tablespoons chopped pimiento (optional)

Mix marinade together. Toss green beans and artichoke hearts in marinade. Keep in a covered glass dish in the refrigerator until ready to cook.

Drain off as much of the marinade as possible. Heat 1 tablespoon olive oil in a large skillet. Toss beans and artichoke hearts until heated through (about 3 or 4 minutes). Add parsley and chives. You can add

2 tablespoons chopped pimiento for color at the last minute. Serve immediately with the poached haddock.

3 protein blocks per serving

LAMB WITH GARLIC CHEESE AND VEGETABLE "PASTA"
(Serves 4)

8 loin lamb chops
2 teaspoons olive oil
1 cup dry red wine
3 garlic cloves, baked
1 tablespoon unsalted butter
1 ounce goat cheese or Rondelé light cheese
Chopped parsley from 6 sprigs. Reserve 4 sprigs for garnish

Trim the fat off the chops and skewer to keep them together to cook more evenly. In a heavy skillet (enameled cast iron or heavy stainless steel), heat the oil very hot. Cook the chops in two batches. Brown the first side, turn over, and salt the seared side. Cook the other side, until the chops are medium rare. Remove to a plate. Cook the remaining chops and remove to a plate.

Pour off the fat and add the red wine. Cook over medium heat until the wine has slowly reduced by half. Press the baked garlic cloves through a small strainer, and add them to the skillet with the butter. Whisk for a moment to emulsify the butter into the sauce.

Taste it and add salt and pepper if you wish. Serve two chops per person with some sauce, and add the juice from the plate. Top with goat or Rondelé cheese. Sprinkle with finely chopped parsley and garnish with parsley sprigs. Serve with Vegetable "Pasta."

VEGETABLE "PASTA"
(Serves 4)

Yellow squash and zucchini, peeled into long shreds with a potato peeler, make a nice change to use like pasta with your chicken or lamb dishes.

2 to 3 medium-sized zucchini*
2 to 3 medium-sized yellow squash*
2 to 3 medium-sized carrots
1 tablespoon butter or olive oil
¼ cup chopped basil
¼ cup chopped parsley
Salt
Freshly ground pepper
Fresh herbs such as basil or dried herbs

Wash the zucchini and the squash. Wash and peel the carrots. With a vegetable peeler, slice the zucchini and squash into long strips. Shred the carrots with a potato peeler into long shreds, and then discard the center core of the carrot. Set aside until ready to cook.

Over medium heat in a large, heavy stainless-steel skillet or a wok heat the butter or oil. Add the shreds. Cook the carrot first, for 2 to 3 minutes, then add the squash and zucchini and toss frequently, cooking for 3 to 4 minutes. (Note: Olive oil allows you to heat the skillet to a higher temperature.) Add salt, pepper, and chopped herbs. Serve immediately with lamb chops.

4 protein blocks per serving

MEXICAN BROILED SWORDFISH WITH MEXICAN HOLIDAY SALAD
(Serves 4)

Marinade:
1 small onion (chopped)
1 clove garlic (mashed or chopped fine)
⅓ cup lime juice
8–12 slices pickled jalapeño pepper
½ cup chopped cilantro
1 tablespoon olive oil

---

*Use only tender zucchini and yellow squash. The centers may be put into a soup.

2 cups water
1½ pounds swordfish fillets cut into 3 eight-ounce portions (¾ to 1
   inch thick)

Place the fillets on the bottom of a glass baking dish (13 by 9 by 2
inches). In a separate glass bowl, mix the marinade ingredients, and
pour the mixture over the fish. Turn the pieces over to ensure that
each piece is coated. Cover the dish and refrigerate for at least one
hour, or marinate overnight for the best flavor.

To cook the fillets: Remove them from the marinade and brush
off any peppers or spices, as these will burn when grilling and taste
bitter. Spray the cold grill with olive-oil spray, and heat to medium
hot. Cook fillets to medium, about 4 minutes per side. If you like
them well done, cook about 5 or 6 minutes per side. Serve at once
with Mexican Holiday Salad.

MEXICAN HOLIDAY SALAD
(Serves 4)

Fresh head lettuce (iceberg or romaine)
Sliced beets (16-ounce can)
2 oranges
1 jícama
½ cup lime juice
2 red apples
Pineapple rings (20-ounce can)
2 bananas
½ cup raw Spanish peanuts

Dressing:
Light mayonnaise
Juice from pineapple

Wash lettuce leaves and separate. Place whole leaves on a large,
round serving dish (14 by 16 inches). Arrange drained beets as an outside ring on top of lettuce.

Peel oranges and remove white membrane. Slice oranges crosswise (like wagon wheels). Peel jícama and cut into thin slices. Dip the slices into the lime juice. Alternate the orange slices with the jícama slices as a ring inside the ring of beets.

Core apples but do not peel. Slice into thin rings. Dip slices into lime juice. Drain pineapple rings, reserving juice in a bowl or measuring cup. Alternate apple rings with pineapple rings inside the orange-and-jícama ring.

Peel bananas and slice into ½-inch slices. Dip into lime juice. Arrange banana slices in center of salad.

Sprinkle bananas with Spanish peanuts.

Mix equal amounts of mayonnaise and pineapple juice. Drizzle over entire salad minutes before serving with swordfish. The arranged salad will keep in the refrigerator about one hour.

(Note: For an elegant variation, Coconut Bananas can be added to the center. To make Coconut Bananas, dip banana slices one at a time in lime juice, then shake off excess. Roll slices in sour cream or yogurt. Then roll in unsweetened shredded coconut. These are delicious!) Serve with Mexican Broiled Swordfish.

4 protein blocks per serving

CHEESE OMELET
(Serves 1)

1 whole egg and 3 egg whites, or 1 cup Egg Beaters
Salt, and freshly cracked white pepper
Olive-oil spray
1 ounce Alpine cheddar cheese
Parsley or cilantro sprig
½ cup chopped tomato, or ¼ cup picante sauce

In a glass measuring cup, whisk the eggs until light in color; add salt and pepper. Spray a skillet with the olive oil, and heat the skillet over medium heat. Pour the egg mixture into the skillet when it is hot, and let cook about 30 seconds. Lift the edge of the omelet with a spatula and let liquid eggs run around the outside. Continue cooking until moist but not runny. Sprinkle cheese in the center of the omelet.

Fold the omelet into thirds and transfer it to a plate.

Garnish with a parsley sprig and freshly chopped tomato or with picante sauce and freshly chopped cilantro.

Serve with 2 pieces of whole rye toast and almond butter.

4 protein blocks per serving

TUNA, ARTICHOKE, AND GREEN-BEAN PASTA SALAD
(Serves about 8)

Vinaigrette dressing:
Salt and freshly cracked pepper
¼ cup red wine vinegar
¼ cup walnut oil
¼ cup olive oil
½ cup parsley, finely chopped
¼ cup chives, finely chopped

18 ounces cut green beans (fresh or frozen), cooked
4 cups bamboo shoots, drained and rinsed in cold water
4 cups water chestnuts, sliced, drained
1 can artichoke hearts, drained
4 cups cooked spiral pasta
24 ounces tuna canned in water
1 head Boston lettuce
Chopped parsley

In a glass bowl or measuring cup, add the salt and pepper to the vinegar and stir until the salt dissolves. Add the other ingredients and stir until well mixed. Set vinaigrette aside.

Cook the beans in the microwave until just tender, 6 to 8 minutes. Drain the bamboo shoots, water chestnuts, and artichoke hearts in a colander, and rinse under cold water. Drain and set aside. Cook pasta according to package directions and rinse with cold water. Drain and measure out 4 cups. Drain the tuna and break up.

In a large bowl, stir the vegetables, pasta, tuna, and vinaigrette dressing until all of the ingredients are coated. Let it marinate in the refrigerator for at least one hour.

To serve, arrange the salad on a platter lined with Boston lettuce and sprinkle it with fresh chopped parsley. Drizzle any remaining dressing on top of the salad.

3 protein blocks per serving

GUACAMOLE

Fajitas are an excellent way to make easy Zone-favorable meals, and a great way of adding monounsaturated fat (like guacamole) to your meals. So let's start with a recipe for guacamole.

1 ripe avocado
Lemon juice
Salt and freshly ground white pepper

Buy a nice ripe avocado, free of bruises. To ripen an avocado, place it in a paper bag for a day or two.

Cut the avocado in half lengthwise, and remove the peel and pit. In a glass bowl, mash the avocado with the lemon juice, salt, and pepper until it is smooth.

Cover and refrigerate it until ready to use. (Optional: You may add some chopped tomato and onion if you wish.)

2 fat blocks per tablespoon

SHRIMP FAJITAS
(Serves 4)

1 pound fresh shrimp (32–40), peeled
6 tablespoons bottled lime juice
Salt and pepper
1 green pepper, cut into 4 even quarters, seeds and membranes
   removed
1 red pepper, cut into 4 even quarters, seeds and membranes
   removed

1 yellow onion, sliced in ¼-inch-wide rings, and microwaved on
   high for 2 minutes, stirring after 1 minute
1½ tablespoons olive oil
4 fajita-style tortillas (8-inch diameter)

Condiments:
2 cups chopped, seeded tomato (½ cup per serving)
½ cup salsa (2 tablespoons per serving)
½ cup guacamole (2 tablespoons per serving)

Put the uncooked shrimp, lime juice, salt and pepper, and enough
water to cover in a glass dish. Cover with a plastic wrap and refrigerate for 3 hours or overnight.

Remove the shrimp from the dish. In a large skillet, over high
heat, add the olive oil, the liquid from the shrimp and cook to reduce
by half. Add the peppers and onion and cook for 3–4 minutes. Add
the shrimp and toss only long enough to warm the shrimp. Do not
overcook them! Remove from the heat and serve immediately with
condiments and tortillas.

3 protein blocks per serving

CHICKEN FAJITAS
(Serves 4)

12 ounces boneless chicken breasts
6 tablespoons bottled lime juice
Salt and freshly ground pepper
¼ cup water or more
1 green pepper, cut into 4 even quarters, seeds and membranes
   removed
1 red pepper, cut into 4 even quarters, seeds and membranes
   removed
1 yellow onion, sliced in ¼-inch-wide rings, and microwaved on
   high for 2 minutes, stirring after 1 minute.
4 fajita-size tortillas (approximately 8-inch diameter)

Condiments (per person):
½ cup chopped tomato
2 tablespoons salsa
2 tablespoons guacamole

Slice chicken breasts crosswise into ½-inch strips. Place in a glass dish with salsa, lime juice, salt, and pepper and enough water to cover. Cover with plastic wrap and refrigerate overnight.

Into a large skillet, over high heat, pour in the liquid from the chicken and cook to reduce by half. Add the chicken strips and, using a large Chinese-type spatula, or wide wooden spatula, toss frequently. When the chicken turns white (opaque) but is not yet thoroughly cooked, add the peppers and onion. Continue cooking by tossing the mixture, and cook until the liquid has evaporated and it begins to sizzle. Give one more toss and remove from heat. Serve with condiments and tortillas.

3 protein blocks per serving

SALMON MOUSSE WITH CUCUMBER SALAD
(Serves 5)

1 16-ounce can red or pink salmon
3 ounces low-fat cream cheese
1 package unflavored gelatin
1 tablespoon chopped fresh dill
Boston lettuce
Black olives

Drain off the salmon juice and clean the salmon by removing the skin and bones. Place the salmon and cream cheese in a food-processor bowl, fitted with the steel blade. Process to mix.

Meanwhile, in a small bowl, sprinkle the gelatin over ¼ cup cold water. Microwave on high (full power) for 30 to 40 seconds, until nicely dissolved. Add it to the salmon mixture and pulse to mix; add the dill, and pulse on/off.

Spoon the mousse into a small fish mold, or other mold, sprayed with olive oil. Pack it in, pressing gently to prevent air bubbles. Cover with plastic wrap and refrigerate for 3 hours or overnight.

Line a fish serving platter with Boston lettuce and unmold the mousse. Place two black olive pieces for the eyes. Serve with Cucumber Salad.

CUCUMBER SALAD
(Makes about four 2-cup servings)

6 cucumbers

1 ½ cups cider vinegar

2 ½ cups warm water

⅓ cup sugar

4 tablespoons salt

2 tablespoons mustard

3 tablespoons dill seed

4 pint-size wide-mouthed
   pickling jars

Wash cucumbers thoroughly with a vegetable brush. Slice as thin as possible. (A food processor with the thinnest slicing blade makes this part go very quickly.)

Mix vinegar, warm water, sugar, salt, and mustard together until sugar and mustard are completely dissolved.

Layer cucumber slices on bottoms of jars. Sprinkle sparingly with dill seed. Continue alternating layers of cucumber slices and dill seeds until jars are nearly full. Pour 1 cup liquid into each jar. Add water to each jar if needed until cucumber slices are covered. Seal jars and refrigerate. Can be eaten in 24 hours. Will keep in the refrigerator for 2 to 3 weeks. Use 2 cups of cucumber salad with each serving of salmon mousse.

3 protein blocks per serving

LESS THAN GOURMET COOKING IN THE ZONE

Obviously gourmet cooking takes time, which is always your greatest obstacle to following a Zone-favorable diet. To help solve that problem, Envion International, Inc., located in Nashua, N.H., has devised an ingenious computer program based on my food-block program to generate several weeks of menus based on the number of protein blocks an individual requires for each meal. It is almost as if you go into a restaurant and order a Zone-favorable meal designed specifically for you, as each meal is exactly scaled to the number of protein blocks you require, but more importantly based upon the meals you would normally find in a restaurant. Usually women will need 3 protein blocks per meal, whereas men will usually require 4. Listed below are some of these computer-generated Zone-favorable meals, each containing 4 blocks of protein.

BREAKFAST CHOICES

Breakfast Quesadilla
1 flour tortilla (6-inch)
2 ounces of shredded low-fat Monterey Jack cheese
2 ounces chopped extra-lean Canadian bacon or ham with chopped scallions, green pepper, and tomato
2 tablespoons of guacamole
1 cup of grapes as a side dish

Old-fashioned Oatmeal
⅔ cup cooked oatmeal sprinkled with nutmeg and cinnamon
3 teaspoons slivered almonds
1 cup low-fat (1 percent) milk
3 ounces extra-lean Canadian bacon

½ cup blueberries as a side dish

Huevos Rancheros
1 whole egg
2 egg whites with chopped onion, green pepper, tomato, chili powder, and cilantro
2 ounces low-fat cheese
1 slice whole-grain bread
1⅓ teaspoons almond butter
1 cup honeydew melon cut into cubes as side dish

Vegetarian Oatmeal
⅔ cup cooked oatmeal sprinkled with nutmeg and cinnamon
1 tablespoon protein powder
1 cup soy milk

⅜ cup unsweetened
applesauce
4 soy sausage links
½ slice whole-grain
bread
2 teaspoons old-fashioned
natural peanut butter

Scrambled Eggs Florentine
1 whole egg
4 egg whites mixed with
chopped onions and
mushrooms
1⅓ cups sautéed spinach
1 ounce shredded low-fat
mozzarella cheese
1 cup of light canned fruit
cocktail as side dish

Bagel and Lox
1 plain bagel
3 ounces lox or smoked
salmon
3 tablespoons of light
cream cheese

Vegetarian Sausage Melt
1 whole-grain English
muffin topped and
broiled with 1½
soy-sausage patties
1 ounce low-fat cheese
1⅓ teaspoons of butter

LUNCH CHOICES

BLT Sandwich
1 slice whole-grain
bread
2 ounces extra-lean
Canadian bacon with
lettuce, tomato slice, and
dill pickle wedge
1 ounce low-fat cheese
½ cup plain low-fat yogurt
with ⅓ cup canned
peaches as dessert

Tuna-Salad Sandwich
1 mini pita pocket
4 ounces tuna packed in
water and drained, with

lettuce, tomato slice, and
1 dill pickle wedge
4 teaspoons light
mayonnaise
1 cup grapes as dessert

"Eggless" Egg-Salad Plate
9 ounces cooked, cooled,
and mashed tofu with
chopped scallions,
parsley, paprika, and
garlic salt
4 teaspoons light
mayonnaise
1 pita pocket with lettuce
and tomato slice

½ cup plain low-fat yogurt
1 peach as dessert

Grilled Chicken Caesar Salad
4 ounces shredded grilled
chicken breast served on
top of a large tossed
salad
1 tablespoon caesar
dressing
2 teaspoons olive oil and
vinegar dressing
½ bread stick
1 apple as dessert

Vegetarian Burger
1 soy burger patty
½ ounce low-fat cheese
½ hamburger roll, with
lettuce, tomato slice, and
dill pickle wedge
1 large tossed salad
4 teaspoons
olive-oil-and-vinegar
dressing
¼ cup low-fat cottage
cheese
1 plum as dessert

Chili
4½ ounces lean ground
meat (beef or turkey).
Brown meat with minced
onions, chopped
mushrooms, green
peppers, chili powder,
oregano, and salt with:
1⅓ teaspoons olive oil
½ can kidney beans
1½ cups crushed canned
tomatoes.
Simmer 30 minutes until
beans are tender. Top
with:
1 ounce shredded low-
fat Monterey Jack
cheese

Seafood Salad
6 ounces shrimp, lobster,
or crabmeat with
chopped celery and
onions
4 teaspoons light
mayonnaise
1 large tossed salad
1 carrot cut into sticks
½ mini pita pocket
½ orange as dessert

DINNER CHOICES

Pork Medallion and Apples
4 ounces sautéed pork
medallions with
rosemary, Dijon

mustard, and 2 teaspoons
white wine
1 sliced apple
1¼ cups steamed broccoli

1 large tossed salad
4 teaspoons of
   olive oil-and-vinegar
   dressing

Broiled Lemon Salmon

6 ounces broiled salmon
   fillet with lemon and
   mushroom slices
1 broiled tomato cut in half
   and sprinkled with 1
   teaspoon grated
   Parmesan cheese
1 cup steamed green beans
1 large spinach salad
4 teaspoons of
   olive oil-and-vinegar
   dressing
½ cup red grapes as dessert

Ginger Chicken Stir-fry

4 ounces chicken breast cut
   into strips, with chopped
   onions, red and green
   peppers, mushrooms,
   and grated ginger
1¼ cups chopped broccoli
1¼ cups chopped
   cauliflower
¾ cup snow peas
1⅓ teaspoons peanut oil
1 cup strawberries as
   dessert

Veal Paprika

4 ounces lean scallops of
   veal pounded thin.
   Brown the veal with

slices of onion in
vegetable-oil cooking
spray. Season with
paprika, garlic powder,
cayenne, and salt. Add
vermouth and simmer
over low heat until
tender.
1⅓ cups steamed spinach
1 large tossed salad
4 tablespoons
   olive oil-and-vinegar
   dressing
1 apple as dessert

Tofu Stir-fry

12 ounces tofu cut into
   cubes, with chopped
   onion, red and green
   peppers, mushrooms,
   and soy sauce
2½ cups chopped broccoli
¾ cup snow peas
1⅓ teaspoons peanut oil
⅓ cup of water
1 cup cubed cantaloupe as
   dessert

Shrimp Scampi

5 ounces shrimp sautéed
   with chopped onion,
   green pepper, garlic, and
   salt in ⅓ cup dry white
   wine and 1 teaspoon of
   lemon juice
2½ cups steamed broccoli
1 large tossed salad
4 teaspoons olive oil-

and-vinegar dressing
1 orange as dessert

Curried Chicken
    4 ounces sautéed chicken
      breast with chopped
      garlic, onions, and
      peppers

1 tomato cut into wedges
1 cup green beans
1 large tossed salad
4 teaspoons olive oil-
    and-vinegar dressing
½ cup grapes as dessert

REAL-LIFE COOKING

Obviously not everyone is a cook, including me. In fact, most of my cooking techniques involve turning a microwave oven on and off. So here are some frozen convenience meals that can be found in most supermarkets and that are reasonably Zone-favorable alone as purchased.

Lean Cuisine
    Homestyle Turkey with Vegetables *(3 protein blocks)*
    Chicken in Peanut Sauce *(3 protein blocks)*
    Chicken Oriental with Vegetables *(3 protein blocks)*

Healthy Choice
    Glazed Chicken Breast *(3 protein blocks)*
    Homestyle Classics Barbecue Ribs *(4 protein blocks)*

Budget Gourmet
    Light and Healthy Turkey Dinner *(3 protein blocks)*

Weight Watchers
    Lasagne *(3 protein blocks)*

Virtually any frozen convenience meal can be made into a Zone-favorable meal with the appropriate addition of either additional protein (if the convenience meal contains too many carbohydrate blocks relative to the number of protein blocks) or by adding additional vegetables or fruits (if the convenience meal contains too many protein blocks relative to the number of carbohydrate blocks). With the appropriate additions, you now have a Zone-favorable convenience meal. The following is not meant to be an exhaustive list by any means, only showing that with some simple adjustments any meal can become a Zone-favorable meal. However, do keep in mind that frozen convenience meals are notoriously low in micronutrients.

Turkey-based Meals

Le Menu—Light Traditional Turkey, with ⅓ cup peas, small garden salad with 1 tablespoon Italian dressing. *(3 protein blocks)*

Lean Cuisine—Turkey Dijon, with 1 cup steamed broccoli. *(4 protein blocks)*

Beef-based Meals

Lean Cuisine—Meat Lasagne, with 1 cup steamed broccoli and 1 apple. *(4 protein blocks)*

Lean Cuisine—Beef Szechwan and Noodles, with ½ cup green beans. *(3 protein blocks)*

Budget Gourmet—Light and Healthy Roast Beef, with a side salad with 1 tablespoon olive oil–based dressing and ½ cup strawberries. *(4 protein blocks)*

Le Menu—Beef Sirloin Tips, with ½ cup of broccoli and ½ cup of cantaloupe. *(5 protein blocks)*

Hormel—Beef Stew with side salad and 1 tablespoon Italian dressing. *(3 protein blocks)*

Chicken-based Meals

Stouffer's—Chicken Cacciatore, with tossed green salad and 1 tablespoon olive oil-and-vinegar dressing. *(4 protein blocks)*

Lean Cuisine—Chicken Breast in Herb Sauce, with 1 cup of broccoli and an orange and 1 pat almond butter. *(5 protein blocks)*

Budget Gourmet—Light and Healthy Chicken Breast with Fettucine, with 1 cup broccoli and 1 pat almond butter. *(4 protein blocks)*

Lean Cuisine—Cantonese-style Shrimp and Chicken, with 1 cup of broccoli. *(4 protein blocks)*

Fish-based Meals
> Lean Cuisine—Fish Divan, with tossed salad, 1 tablespoon olive oil-and-vinegar dressing, and an apple. *(5 protein blocks)*
> Lean Cuisine—Fish Filet Jardinière, with 1 cup green beans, side salad, and 1 tablespoon of French dressing. *(4 protein blocks)*

FAST FOOD IN THE ZONE

Okay, if even turning on the microwave is too tough for you, then you can still get relatively Zone-favorable meals in fast-food restaurants. Fast-food choices will tend to be higher in fat than desired (especially if they are hamburgers), but that's what you get for true convenience. Chicken-based meals will always be lower in fat than beef-based meals. Of course, forget the possibility of any micronutrients. Here is a selected listing.

Burger King
> BK Broiler Chicken Sandwich *(3 protein blocks)*
> Plain hamburger *(3 protein blocks)*

Jack in the Box
> Chicken Fajita Pita *(3 protein blocks)*

Hardee's
> Grilled Chicken Sandwich *(3 protein blocks)*

McDonald's
> McGrilled Chicken Sandwich *(3 protein blocks)*
> McLean Deluxe (without cheese) *(3 protein blocks)*
> Egg McMuffin *(2 protein blocks)*
> Two small regular hamburgers
>   (combine the patties and throw
>   away one of the buns) *(3 protein blocks)*

Taco Bell
> Soft chicken taco *(2 protein blocks)*

Wendy's
  Grilled Chicken Sandwich *(4 protein blocks)*
  Chili *(3 protein blocks)*
  Plain hamburger *(3 protein blocks)*

REALLY QUICK MEALS

Don't have time even to go to the fast-food restaurant? Try some of these very quick meals at home.

Breakfast
  1⅓ cups cooked oatmeal with 1 cup low-fat cottage cheese *(4 protein blocks)*
  1 cup cooked oatmeal fortified with 2 tablespoons (1 ounce) protein powder (always add the protein powder after cooking the oatmeal) *(4 protein blocks)*
  4-"egg" omelet (4 egg whites) and 2 cups strawberries *(2 protein blocks)*

Lunch
  4 ounces turkey breast or tuna with 1 teaspoon mayonnaise, and 2 pieces of whole-rye bread *(4 protein blocks)*

Dinner
  4 ounces chicken breast, 1 cup cooked broccoli, 1 orange, and a large dinner salad with 1 tablespoon olive oil-and-vinegar dressing *(4 protein blocks)*

SNACKS

Snacks are a very important aspect of the success of a Zone-favorable diet, in that they allow you never to go more than five hours without a Zone-favorable meal. Listed below are some of the simple snacks that have the correct macronutrient combinations.

PROTEIN-FORTIFIED CORNBREAD MUFFINS

1 package Jiffy Corn Muffin mix (6 ounces)
7 tablespoons protein powder
2 eggs or 1 cup egg substitute
1 cup low-fat milk
1 tablespoon olive oil

Blend the ingredients together, and fill individual foil-lined muffin cups half full. Bake at 300 degrees for 35–40 minutes. Makes approximately 20 muffins. *(1 protein block per muffin)*

CHOCOLATE MALT
(Serves 3)

½ cup low-fat ice cream
½ cup low-fat milk
2 tablespoons protein powder
½ teaspoon Nestlé's sugar-free cocoa

Mix ingredients in high-speed blender. *(1 protein block per serving)*

Cottage cheese and fruit is also a good choice, as is plain yogurt:

—¼ cup low-fat cottage cheese and ½ piece of fruit *(1 protein block)*
—1 cup low-fat yogurt without any added fruit or carbohydrates *(1 protein block)*

GUILTLESS PLEASURES

Even the most delicious carbohydrate-rich dessert can be indulged in with the addition of the appropriate amount of protein. Consider it eicosanoid "damage control," but just don't do it very often.

—½ cup Häagen-Dazs ice cream plus 1 cup low-fat cottage cheese or 4 ounces sliced turkey *(4 protein blocks)*

—1 Snickers bar plus ⅔ cup low-fat cottage cheese or 3 ounces sliced turkey *(3 protein blocks)*

—12-ounce bottle beer plus ½ cup low-fat cottage cheese or 2 ounces sliced turkey *(2 protein blocks)*

—1 small piece Boston cream pie plus 1 cup low-fat cottage cheese or 4 ounces sliced turkey *(4 protein blocks)*

CALCULATION OF YOUR DAILY PROTEIN REQUIREMENTS

1. Determine your lean body mass by consulting Appendix B.
2. Determine your activity factor. Factors are listed below in grams of protein per pound of lean body mass.

> 0.5 - Sedentary (no formal sports activity or training)
> 0.6 - Light fitness training, such as walking
> 0.7 - Moderate training (3 times a week) or sports participation
> 0.8 - Daily aerobic training or daily moderate weight training
> 0.9 - Heavy daily weight training
> 1.0 - Heavy daily weight training coupled with intense sports training or twice-a-day intense sports training

3. Finally, calculate your required daily amount of protein (in grams): multiply your lean body mass (in lbs.) by your activity factor.

The following table will give you representative protein requirements based on lean body mass and activity factors.

LEAN BODY MASS (IN LBS.)	ACTIVITY FACTOR (GRAMS OF PROTEIN PER POUND OF LEAN BODY MASS)					
	0.5	0.6	0.7	0.8	0.9	1.0
90	45	54	63	72	81	90
100	50	60	70	80	90	100
110	55	66	77	88	99	110
120	60	72	84	96	108	120
130	65	78	91	104	117	130
140	70	84	98	112	126	140
150	75	90	105	120	135	150
160	80	96	112	128	144	160
170	85	102	119	136	153	170
180	90	108	126	144	162	180
190	95	114	133	152	171	190
200	100	120	140	160	180	200
210	105	126	147	168	189	210
220	110	132	154	176	198	220
230	115	138	161	184	207	230
240	120	144	168	192	216	240

COMPARISON OF BODY-FAT PERCENTAGES

Your percentage of body fat is the most important measurement you have to determine your progress toward physical fitness. However, to have relevance, this number must have some relationship to real-life situations. Below is a listing of body-fat percentages for elite athletes that will allow you to put your percent of body fat into a better perspective. It is important to note two items. First, males will always have a lower percent of body fat than females in the same reference groups. Second, the reference groups are those for world-class or professional athletes. To have the look of a world-class athlete you have to have the same percentage of body fat as a world-class athlete. But before you can have the look of a world-class athlete, you have to first get to percent body fat for healthy, ideal fit male or female.

REFERENCE GROUP—MALES	PERCENT BODY FAT
Gymnasts, wrestlers	4
Body builders	5
Basketball centers	7
Cross-country skiers, triathletes	8
Racquetball players	9
Basketball forwards, soccer players	10
Swimmers	10
Distance runners, football defensive backs	11
Basketball guards, football linebackers	12
Football offensive backs	13
Ideal male	15
Power lifters, shot putters, discus throwers	17
Average American male	23

REFERENCE GROUP—FEMALES	PERCENT BODY FAT
Average anorexic patient	10
Gymnasts	14
Racquetball players	15
Aerobic-dancer instructors	17
Cross-country skiers	18
Swimmers	19
Tennis players, alpine skiers	20
Track and field, basketball, and volleyball players	21
Ideal female	22
Average American female	32

METROPOLITAN LIFE TABLES FOR IDEAL BODY WEIGHT, 1959 vs. 1983

Height is measured in bare feet, and weight without any clothes. The numbers in parentheses are the 1959 ideal body weights, the **bold-face** numbers are the 1983 ideal body weights. Note the large increases for women.

Men

HEIGHT	SMALL FRAME	MEDIUM FRAME	LARGE FRAME
5'1"	**123–134** (107–115)	**126–136** (113–124)	**133–145** (121–136)
5'2"	**125–131** (110–118)	**128–138** (116–128)	**135–148** (124–139)
5'3"	**127–133** (113–121)	**130–140** (119–131)	**137–151** (127–143)
5'4"	**129–135** (116–124)	**132–143** (122–134)	**139–155** (131–147)
5'5"	**131–137** (119–128)	**134–146** (125–138)	**141–159** (133–151)
5'6"	**133–140** (123–132)	**137–149** (129–142)	**145–163** (137–156)
5'7"	**135–143** (127–136)	**140–152** (133–147)	**147–167** (142–161)
5'8"	**137–145** (131–140)	**143–155** (137–151)	**150–171** (146–165)
5'9"	**139–149** (135–145)	**146–158** (141–155)	**153–175** (150–169)
5'10"	**141–152** (139–149)	**149–161** (145–160)	**156–179** (154–174)
5'11"	**144–155** (143–153)	**152–165** (149–165)	**159–183** (159–179)
6'	**147–159** (147–157)	**155–169** (153–170)	**163–187** (163–184)
6'1"	**150–163** (151–162)	**159–173** (157–175)	**167–192** (168–189)
6'2"	**153–167** (155–166)	**162–177** (162–180)	**171–197** (173–194)
6'3"	**157–171** (159–170)	**166–182** (167–185)	**176–202** (177–199)

Women

HEIGHT	SMALL FRAME	MEDIUM FRAME	LARGE FRAME
4'9"	**99–108** (89–95)	**106–118** (93–104)	**115–128** (101–116)
4'10"	**100–110** (91–98)	**108–120** (95–107)	**117–131** (103–119)
4'11"	**101–112** (93–101)	**110–123** (98–110)	**119–134** (106–122)
5'	**103–115** (96–104)	**112–126** (101–113)	**122–137** (109–125)
5'1"	**105–118** (99–107)	**116–129** (104–116)	**125–140** (112–128)
5'2"	**108–121** (102–110)	**118–132** (107–119)	**128–144** (115–131)
5'3"	**111–124** (105–113)	**121–135** (110–123)	**131–148** (118–135)
5'4"	**114–127** (108–116)	**124–138** (113–127)	**134–152** (122–139)
5'5"	**117–130** (111–120)	**127–141** (117–132)	**137–156** (126–143)
5'6"	**120–133** (115–124)	**130–144** (121–136)	**140–160** (130–147)
5'7"	**123–136** (119–128)	**133–147** (125–140)	**143–164** (134–151)
5'8"	**126–139** (123–132)	**136–150** (129–144)	**146–167** (138–155)
5'9"	**129–142** (127–137)	**139–153** (133–148)	**149–170** (142–160)
5'10"	**132–145** (131–141)	**142–156** (137–152)	**152–173** (146–165)
5'11"	**135–148** (135–145)	**145–159** (141–156)	**155–176** (150–170)

GLYCEMIC INDEX OF CARBOHYDRATES

Rapid inducers of insulin

Glycemic index greater than 100%
  Grain-based foods
      Puffed rice
      Corn flakes
      Puffed wheat
      Millet
      Instant rice
      Instant potato
      Microwaved potato
      French bread
  Simple sugars
      Maltose
      Glucose
  Snacks
      Tofu ice cream
      Puffed-rice cakes
Glycemic index standard = 100%
  White bread
Glycemic index between 80 and 100%
Grain-based foods
      Grapenuts
      Whole-wheat bread
      Rolled oats
      Oat bran
      Instant mashed potatoes
      White rice

Brown rice
Muesli
Shredded wheat
Vegetables
   Carrots
   Parsnips
   Corn
Fruits
   Banana
   Raisins
   Apricots
   Papaya
   Mango
Snacks
   Ice cream (low-fat)
   Corn chips
   Rye crisps

Moderate inducers of insulin
Glycemic index between 50 and 80%
   Grain-based foods
      Spaghetti (white)
      Spaghetti (whole wheat)
      Pasta, other
      Pumpernickel bread
      All-bran cereal
   Fruits
      Orange
      Orange juice
   Vegetables
      Peas
      Pinto beans
      Garbanzo beans
      Kidney beans (canned)
      Baked beans

Navy beans
Simple sugars
    Lactose
    Sucrose
Snacks
    Candy bar*
    Potato chips (with fat)*

Reduced insulin secretion

Glycemic index between 30 and 50%
    Grain-based foods
        Barley
        Oatmeal (slow-cooking)
        Whole-grain rye bread
    Fruits
        Apple
        Apple juice
        Applesauce
        Pears
        Grapes
        Peaches
    Vegetables
        Kidney beans
        Lentils
        Black-eyed peas
        Chick-peas
        Kidney beans (dried)
        Lima beans
        Tomato soup
        Peas
    Dairy products
        Ice cream (high-fat)*
        Milk (skim)
        Milk (whole)
        Yogurt

Glycemic index 30% or less
   Fruits
      Cherries
      Plums
      Grapefruit
   Simple sugars
      Fructose
   Vegetables
      Soy beans*
   Snacks
      Peanuts*

---

*High fat content will retard the rate of absorption of carbohydrate into the body.

BIBLIOGRAPHY

INTRODUCTION

Adams, C. W. M., Y. H. Abdulla, O. B. Bayliss, and R. S. Morgan. "Modification of aortic atheroma and fatty liver in cholesterol-free rabbits by intravenous injection of saturated and polyunsaturated lecithins." *Journal of Pathological Bacteria* (1967) 94: 77–87.

Altman, R. F. A., J. M. de Mendonca, G. M. V. Schaeffer, J. Ramos de Souza, J. G. Bandoli, D. J. Silva, and C. R. N. Lopes. "Phospholipids in experimental atherosclerosis." Arzeim-Frosch. *(Drug Research)* (1974) 24: 11–16.

Byers, S. O., and M. Friedman. "Effect of infusion of phosphatides upon atherosclerotic aorta in situ and as an ocular aortic implant." *Journal of Lipid Research* (1960) 1: 343–348.

Campannacci, L., G. Guarnieri, L. Faccine, and G. Bellini. "Response of plasma lipid fractions to administration of exogenous phospholipids." *Drug Research* (1975) 25: 1306–1308.

Cazzolato, A. P., B. G. Bittolo, G. B. Quinci, F. Belussi, O. Mantero, and F. Conti. "Modification of lipids, lipoproteins and plasma apolipoproteins induced by a phospholipid extracted from calf liver." *Pharmacology Research Communications* (1977) 9: 885–892.

Friedman, M., S. O. Byers, and R. H. Rosenman. "Resolution of aortic atherosclerotic infiltrations in the rabbit by phosphatide infusion." *Proc. Soc. Exp. Biol. Med.* (1957) 95: 586–588.

Howard, A. N., J. Patelski, D. E. Bowyer, and G. A. Gresham. "Atherosclerosis induced in hypercholesterolemic baboons by immunological injury and the effects of intravenous polyunsaturated phosphatidylcholine." *Atherosclerosis* (1971) 14: 17–29.

Maurukas, J., and R. G. Thomas. "Treatment of experimental atherosclerosis in the rabbit with L, D alpha (dimyristoly) lecithin." *Journal of Laboratory and Clinical Medicine* (1960) 55: 30–37.

Patelski, J., D. E. Bowyer, A. N. Howard, I. W. Jennings, C. J. R. Thorne, and G. A. Gresham. "Modification of enzyme activities in experimental atherosclerosis in the rabbit." *Atherosclerosis* (1970) 12: 41–53.

Stafford, W. W., and C. E. Day. "Regression of atherosclerosis effected by intravenous phospholipid." *Artery* (1975) 1: 106–114.

CHAPTER 1: LIFE IN THE ZONE

Books

Pele, with R. L. Fish. *My Life and the Beautiful Game: The Autobiography of Pele*. Garden City, NY: 1977.

Pritikin, N., and P. McGrady. *The Pritikin Program for Diet and Exercise*. New York: Grosset and Dunlap, 1979.

Articles

"Are you eating right?" *Consumer Reports* (1992), pp. 644–651.

CHAPTER 2: THE FATTENING OF AMERICA

Books

Atkins, R. C. *Dr. Atkins' Diet Revolution*. New York: Bantam, 1972.

Bailey, C. *The New Fit or Fat*. Boston: Houghton Mifflin, 1991.

Bernstein, R. K. *Diabetes Type II*. New York: Prentice-Hall Press, 1990.

Erzin, C., and R. E. Kowalski. *The Endocrine Control Diet*. New York: Harper & Row, 1990.

Heller, R. F., and R. F. Heller. *The Carbohydrate Addict's Diet*. New York: Penguin, 1991.

Tarnower, H., and S. S. Baker. *The Complete Scarsdale Medical Diet*. New York: Rawson Wade, 1978.

Articles

Brandes, J. "Insulin-induced overeating in the rat." *Physiology Review* (1977) 18: 1095–1102.

Colditz, G. A. "Economic costs of obesity." *American Journal of Clinical Nutrition* (1992) 55: 503S–507S.

Coulston, A. M., G. C. Liu, and G. M. Reaven. "Plasma, glucose, insulin and lipid responses to high-carbohydrate, low-fat diets in normal humans." *Metabolism* (1983) 32: 52–56.

Kern, P. A., J. M. Ong, B. Soffan, and J. Carty. "The effects of weight loss on the activity and expression of adipose-tissue lipoprotein lipire in very obese individuals." *New England Journal of Medicine* (1990) 322: 1053–1059.

Felig, P., and J. Wahren. "Fuel homeostasis in exercise." *New England Journal of Medicine* (1975) 293: 1078–1084.

Food and Agriculture Organization/World Health Organization. "Energy and protein requirements." *WHO Technical Report* (1985) 724.

Friedman, J. E., and P. W. A. Lemon. "Effect of chronic endurance exercise on retention of dietary protein." *International Journal of Sports Medicine* (1989) 10: 118–223.

Grandjean, A. C. "Macronutrient intake of U.S. athletes compared with the general population and recommendations made to athletes." *American Journal of Clinical Nutrition* (1989) 49: 1070–1076.

Gontzea, I., R. Sutzescu, and S. Damitrache. "The influence of adaptation to physical effort on nitrogen balance in man." *Nutrition Report International* (1975) 11: 231–236.

———. "The influence of muscular activity on nitrogen balance and on need of man for protein." *Nutrition Report International* (1974) 10: 35–39.

Hamm, P., R. B. Shekelle, and J. Stamler. "Large fluctuations in body weight during young adulthood and 25-year risk of coronary death in men." *American Journal of Epidemiology* (1989) 129: 312–318.

Hannon, B. M., and T. G. Lohman. "The energy cost of overweight in the United States." *American Journal of Public Health* (1978) 68: 765–767.

Jenkins, D. J. A., T. M. S. Wolever, and R. H. Taylor. "Glycemic index of foods: a physiological basis for carbohydrate exchange." *American Journal of Clinical Nutrition* (1981) 34: 362–366.

Kaczmarski, R. J., K. M. Flegal, S. M. Comptede, and C. L. Johnson. "Increasing prevalence of overweight among U.S. adults." *Journal of the American Medical Association* (1994) 272: 205–239.

Kanarek, R., R. Marks-Kaufman, and B. Lipeles. "Increased carbohy-

drate intake as a function of insulin administration in rats."
Physiological Behavior (1980) 25: 779–782.

Kekwick, A., and G. L. S. Pawan. "Calorie intake in relation to body-weight changes in the obese." *Lancet* (1956) 2: 155–161.

———. "Metabolic study in human obesity with isocaloric diets high in fat, protein or carbohydrate." *Metabolism* (1957) 6: 447–460.

Laurier, D., M. Guiguet, N. P. Chan, J. A. Wells, and A. J. Valleron. "Prevalence of obesity: a comparative survey in France, the United Kingdom, and the United States." *International Journal of Obesity* (1992) 16: 565–572.

Lee, I. M., and R. S. Paffenbarger. "Change in body weight and longevity." *Journal of the American Medical Association* (1992) 268: 2045–2049.

Lisser, L., P. M. Odell, R. B. D'Agostino, J. Stokes, B. E. Kraeger, M. A. Bellanger, and K. D. Brownell. "Variability of body weight and health outcomes in the Framingham population." *New England Journal of Medicine* (1991) 324: 1839–1844.

Meredith, C. N., M. J. Zockin, W. R. Frontera, and W. J. Evans. "Dietary protein requirements and body protein metabolism in endurance-trained men." *Journal of Applied Physiology* (1989) 66: 2850–2856.

Norman, A. W., and G. Litwack. "Pancreatic Hormones," in *Hormones*. New York: Academic Press, 1987, pp. 264–319.

Sadur, C. N., and R. H. Eckel. "Insulin stimulation of adipose tissue lipoprotein lipase." *Journal of Clinical Investigation* (1982) 69: 1119–1123.

Swisklocki, A. M., Y. D. Chen, M. A. Golay, M. D. Cheng, and G. M. Reaven. "Insulin suppression of plasma-free fatty acid concentration in normal individuals or patients with type II (non-insulin-dependent) diabetes." *Diabetologia* (1987) 30: 622–626.

Wolever, T. M. S. "Relationship between dietary fiber content and composition in foods and the glycemic index." *American Journal of Clinical Nutrition* (1990) 51: 72–75.

Wolever, T. M. S., D. J. A. Jenkins, A. A. Jenkins, and R. G. Josse. "The glycemic index: methodology and clinical implications." *American Journal of Clinical Nutrition* (1991) 54: 846–854.

Young, V. R. "Protein and amino acid requirements in humans." *Scandinavian Journal of Nutrition* (1992) 36: 47–56.

Young, V. R., D. M. Bier, and P. L. Pellett. "A theoretical basis for increasing current estimates of the amino acid requirements in adult men with experimental support." *American Journal of Clinical Nutrition* (1989) 50: 80–92.

Young, V. R., and P. L. Pellett. "Plant protein in relation to human protein and amino acid nutrition." *American Journal of Clinical Nutrition* (1994) 59: 1203S–1212S.

CHAPTER 3: THE HORMONAL EFFECTS OF FOOD

Books

Atkins, R. C. *Dr. Atkins' New Diet Revolution.* New York: M. Evans, 1992.

Bernstein, R. K. *Diabetes Type II.* New York: Prentice-Hall Press, 1990.

Eades, M. *Thin So Fast.* New York: Warner Books, 1989.

Erzin, C., and R. E. Kowalski. *The Endocrine Control Diet.* New York: Harper & Row, 1990.

Heller, R. F., and R. F. Heller. *The Carbohydrate Addict's Diet.* New York: Penguin, 1991.

Norman, A. W., and G. Litwack. *Hormones.* New York: Academic Press, 1987.

Winick, M., ed. *Nutrition and Gastroenterology.* New York: John Wiley, 1980.

Articles

Unger, R. H. "Glucagon and the insulin: glucagon ratio in diabetes and other catabolic illnesses." *Diabetes* (1971) 20: 834–838.

CHAPTER 4: EICOSANOIDS—THE SHORT COURSE

Books

Chakrin, L. W., and D. M. Bailey, eds. *The Leukotrienes.* New York: Academic Press, 1989.

Herman, A. G., P. M. Van Houtle, H. Denolin, and A. Goossons, eds. *Cardiovascular Pharmacology of Prostaglandins.* New York: Raven Press, 1982.

Lands, W. E. M. *Fish and Human Health*. New York: Academic Press, 1986.

Ninneman, J. L. *Prostaglandins, Leukotrienes and the Immune Response*. New York: Cambridge University Press, 1988.

Thaler-Dao, H., A. Crastes de Paulet, and R. Paoletti. *Icosanoids and Cancer*. New York: Raven Press, 1989.

Willis, A. L. *Handbook of Eicosanoids, Prostaglandins and Related Lipids*. Boca Raton, FL: CRC Press, 1987.

Articles

Bergstrom, S., R. Rhyhage, B. Samuelsson, and J. Scorval. "The structure of prostaglandins E_1, E_1a and F_1B." *Journal of Biology and Chemistry* (1963) 238: 3555–3565.

Burr, G. O., and M. R. Burr. "A new deficiency disease produced by rigid exclusion of fat from the diet." *Journal of Biology and Chemistry* (1929) 82: 345–367.

———. "On the nature and role of the fatty acids essential in nutrition." *Journal of Biology and Chemistry* (1930) 86: 587–621.

Hamberg, M., and B. Samuelsson. "Detection and isolation of an endoperoxide intermediate in prostaglandin bysyntheses." *Proceedings of the National Academy of Science USA* (1973) 70: 899–903.

Hamberg, M., J. Svensson, and B. Samuelsson. "Thromboxanes: A new group of biologically active compounds derived from prostaglandin endoperoxides." *Proceedings of the National Academy of Science USA* (1975) 72: 2994–2998.

Hamberg, M., J. Svensson, T. Wakabayashi, and B. Samuelsson. "Isolation and structure of two prostaglandin endoperoxides that cause platelet aggregation." *Proceedings of the National Academy of Science USA* (1974) 71: 345–349.

Johnson, R. A., D. R. Morton, J. A. Kinver, R. R. Gorman, J. C. McGuire, F. F. Sun, N. Whither, S. Bunting, J. Salmon, S. Moncada, and J. R. Vane. "The chemical structure of prostaglandin X (prostacyclin)." *Prostaglandins* (1976) 12: 915–928.

Metz, S., W. Fujimoto, and R. O. Robertson. "Modulation of insulin secretion by cyclic AMP and prostaglandin E." *Metabolism* (1982) 31: 1014–1033.

Metz, S., M. van Rollins, R. Strife, W. Fujimoto, and R. P. Robertson. "Lipoxygenase pathway in islet endrocrine cells—Oxidate metabolism of arachidonic acid promotes insulin release." *Journal of Clinical Investigation* (1983) 71: 1191–1205.

Moncada, S., R. Gryglewsk, S. Bunting, and J. R. Vane. "An enzyme isolated from arteries transforms prostaglandin endoperoxides to an unstable substance that inhibits platelet aggregation." *Nature (London)* (1976) 263: 663–665.

Pek, S. B., and M. F. Walsh. "Leukotrienes stimulate insulin released from rat pancreas." *Proceedings of the National Academy of Science USA* (1984) 82: 2199–2202.

Robertson, R. P. "Prostaglandins, glucose homeostasis and diabetes mellitus." *Annual Review of Medicine* (1983) 34: 1–12.

Robertson, R. P., D. J. Gavarenski, D. Porte, and E. L. Bierman. "Inhibition of in vivo insulin secretion by prostaglandin E_1." *Journal of Clinical Investigation* (1974) 54: 310–315.

Samuelsson, B. "On incorporation of oxygen in the conversion of 8, 11, 14 eicoatrienoic acid into prostaglandin E." *Journal of American Chemical Society* (1965) 89: 3011–3013.

Sears, B. "Essential fatty acids and dietary endocrinology." *Journal of Advanced Medicine* (1993) 6: 211–224.

Serhan, C. N. "Lipoxin biosynthesis and its impact in inflammatory and vascular events." *Biochemistry and Biophysics Acta* (1994) 1212: 1–25.

von Euler, U. S. "On the specific vasodilating and plain muscle stimulating substances from accessory genital glands in men and certain animals (prostaglandins and vesiglandin)." *Journal of Physiology (London)* (1936) 88: 213–234.

CHAPTER 5: ELITE ATHLETES IN THE ZONE

Books

Haas, R. *Eat to Win.* New York: Rawson Associates, 1983.

Viru, A. *Hormones in Muscular Activity.* Boca Raton, FL: CRC Press, 1985.

Articles

Balson, P. D., B. Ekblom, and B. Sjodin. "Enhanced oxygen availability during high intensity intermittent exercise decreases anaerobic metabolite concentrations in blood." *Acta Physiologica Scandinavia* (1994) 150: 455–456.

Chandler, R. M., H. K. Byrne, J. G. Patterson, and J. L. Ivy. "Dietary supplements affect the anabolic hormones after weight-training exercise." *Journal of Applied Physiology* (1994) 76: 839–845.

Crist, D. M., G. T. Peake, P. A. Egan, and D. L. Waters. "Body composition response to exogenous GH during training in highly conditioned adults." *Journal of Applied Physiology* (1988) 65: 579–584.

Ekblom, B., and B. Berglund. "Effect of erythropoietin administration on maximal aerobic power." *Scandinavian Journal of Medical Science in Sports* (1991) 1: 88–93.

Gaitanos, G., C. Williams, L. H. Boobis, and S. Brooks. "Human muscle metabolism during intermittent maximal exercise." *Journal of Applied Physiology* (1993) 75: 712–719.

Lamb, D. R., K. F. Rinehardt, R. L. Bartels, W. M. Sherman, and J. T. Snook. "Dietary carbohydrate and intensity of interval swim training." *American Journal of Clinical Nutrition* (1990) 52: 1058–1063.

Muoio, D. M., J. J. Leddy, P. J. Horvath, A. B. Awad, and D. R. Pendergast. "Effect of dietary fat on metabolic adjustments to maximal VO2 and endurance in runners." *Medical Science of Sports and Exercise* (1994) 26: 81–88.

Phinney, S. D., B. R. Bistrian, W. J. Evans, E. Gervino, and G. L. Blackburn. "The human metabolic response to chronic ketosis without caloric restriction." *Metabolism* (1983) 32: 769–776.

Sherman, W. M., J. A. Doyle, D. R. Lamb, and R. H. Strauss. "Dietary carbohydrate, muscle glycogen and exercise performance during 7d of training." *American Journal of Clinical Nutrition* (1993) 57: 21–31.

Whitten, P. "Stanford's secret weapon." *Swimming World* (1993) 34: 28–33.

Zawadzki, K. M., B. B. Yaspelkis, and J. L. Ivy. "Carbohydrate-protein complex increases the rate of muscle glycogen storage after exercise." *Journal of Applied Physiology* (1992) 72: 1854–1859.

CHAPTER 6: EXERCISE IN THE ZONE

Books

Bailey, C. *The New Fit or Fat.* Boston: Houghton Mifflin, 1991.

———. *Smart Exercise.* Boston: Houghton Mifflin, 1994.

Edwards, S. *The Heart Rate Monitor Book.* Sacramento, CA: Fleet Feet Press, 1992.

Norman, A. W., and G. Litwock. *Hormones.* New York: Academic Press, 1987.

Stanford, B. A., and P. Shimer. *Fitness without Exercise.* New York: Warner Books, 1990.

Viru, A. *Hormones in Muscular Activity.* Boca Raton, FL: CRC Press, 1983.

Articles

Astrom, C., and J. Lindholm. "Growth hormone deficient young adults have decreased deep sleep." *Neuroendocrinology* (1990) 51: 82–84.

Astrom, C., S. A. Petersen, and J. Lindholm. "The influence of growth hormone on sleep in adults with growth hormone deficiencies." *Clinical Endocrinology* (1990) 33: 495–500.

Astrom, C., and W. Trojaboy. "Effect of growth hormone on human sleep energy." *Clinical Endocrinology* (1992) 36: 241–245.

Bak, J. F., N. Moeller, and O. Schmitic. "Effects of growth hormone on fuel utilization and muscle glycogen synthesis activity in normal humans." *American Journal of Physiology* (1991) 260: E736–742.

Chatzipanteli, K., S. Rudolph, and L. Axelrod. "Coordinate control of lipolysis by prostaglandins E_2 and prostacyclin in rat adipose tissue." *Diabetes* (1992) 41: 927–935.

Crist, D. M., G. T. Peake, P. A. Egan, and D. L. Waters. "Body composition response to exogenous GH during training in highly conditioned adults." *Journal of Applied Physiology* (1988) 65: 579–584.

Galbo, H., J. J. Holst, and N. J. Christensen. "The effect of different diets of insulin on the hormonal response to prolonged exercise." *Acta Physiology Scandinavia* (1979) 107: 19–32.

———. "Glucagon and plasma catecholamine response to graded

and prolonged exercise in man." *Journal of Applied Physiology* (1975) 38: 70–76.

Hartman, M. L., P. E. Clayton, M. L. Johnson, et al. "A low-dose euglycemic infusion of recombinant human insulin-like growth factor I rapidly suppresses fasting-enhanced pulsatile growth hormone secretion in humans." *Journal of Clinical Investigation* (1993) 91: 2453–2462.

Janssen, P. G. J. M. "Heart rate monitoring for estimation of training intensity," in *Medicine in Sports Training and Coaching*, edited by P. W. R. Lemon, J. Karvonen, and I. Iliev. Basel, Switzerland: Krager, 1992, pp. 115–159.

Paffenbarger, R. S., A. L. Wing, and R. T. Hyde. "Physical activity as an index of heart attack risk in college alumni." *American Journal of Epidemiology* (1978) 108: 161–175.

Paffenbarger, R. S., R. T. Hyde, A. L. Wing, and C. Hsieh. "Physical activity, all-cause mortality, and longevity of college alumni." *New England Journal of Medicine* (1986) 314: 615–613.

Paffenbarger, R. S., and W. E. Hale. "Work activity and coronary heart mortality." *New England Journal of Medicine* (1970) 292: 1109–1114.

Racette, S. B., D. A. Schoeller, R. F. Kushner, K. M. Neil, and K. Herling-Iaffaldano. "Effects of aerobic exercise and dietary carbohydrate on energy expenditure and body composition during weight reduction in obese women." *American Journal of Clinical Nutrition* (1995) 61: 486–494.

Roth, J., S. M. Gluck, R. S. Yalow, and S. A. Berson. "The influence of blood glucose on the plasma concentration of growth hormone." *Diabetes* (1964) 13: 355–361.

Rudman, D., A. G. Feller, H. S. Hagraj, G. A. Gerhans, P. Y. Lalitha, and A. F. Goldber. "Effects of human growth hormone in men over 60 years old." *New England Journal of Medicine* (1990) 323: 1–6.

Scheele, K., W. Harzog, G. Ruthaler, A. Wirth, and H. Wencher. "Metabolic adaptation to prolonged exercise." *European Journal of Applied Physiology* (1982) 41: 101–106.

Schofield, J. G. "Prostaglandin E_1 and the release of growth hormone in vitro." *Nature* (1970) 228: 179.

Takahoski, Y., D. M. Kipmis, and W. H. Daughaday. "Growth hormone secretion during sleep." *Journal of Clinical Investigation* (1968) 47: 2079–2090.

Weltman, A., J. Y. Weltman, R. Schurrer, W. S. Evans, J. D. Veldhuis, and A. D. Rogal. "Endurance training amplifies the pulsatile release of growth hormone: Effects of training intensity." *Journal of Applied Physiology* (1992) 72: 2188–2196.

Yamashita, S., and S. Melmed. "Effects of insulin on rat anterior pituitary cells: Inhibition of growth hormone secretion and mRNA levels." *Diabetes* (1986) 35: 440–447.

CHAPTER 7: BOUNDARIES OF THE ZONE

Books

Atkins, R. C. *Dr. Atkins' New Diet Revolution.* New York: M. Evans, 1992.

Norman, A. W., and G. Litwack. *Hormones.* New York: Academic Press, 1987.

Articles

Dek, S. B., and M. F. Walsh. "Leukotrienes stimulate insulin release from rat pancreas." *Proceedings of the National Academy of Science USA* (1985) 81: 2199–2202.

Hamm, P., R. B. Shekelle, and J. Stamler. "Large fluctuations in body weight during young adulthood and 25-years risk of coronary death in men." *American Journal of Epidemiology* (1989) 129: 312–318.

Kern, P. A., J. M. Ong, B. Soffan, and J. Carty. "The effects of weight loss on the activity and expression of adipose-tissue lipoprotein lipase in very obese individuals." *New England Journal of Medicine* (1990) 322: 1053–1059.

Lee, I. M., and R. S. Paffenbarger. "Change in body weight and longevity." *Journal of the American Medical Association* (1992) 268: 2045–2049.

Lisser, L., P. M. Odell, R. B. D'Agostino, J. Strokes, B. E. Kreger, A. J. Belanger, and K. D. Brownell. "Variability of body weight and health outcomes in the Framingham population." *New England Journal of Medicine* (1991) 324: 1839–1844.

Sadur, C. N., and R. H. Echel. "Insulin stimulation of adipose tissue lipoprotein lipase." *Journal of Clinical Investigation* (1982) 69: 1119–1123.

Silver, M. J., W. Hoch, J. J. Koesis, C. M. Ingerman, and J. B. Smith. "Arachidonic acid causes sudden death in rabbits." *Science* (1974) 183: 1035–1037.

Simsolo, R. B., J. M. Ong, B. Saffari, and P. A. Kern. "Effect of improved diabetes control on the expression of lipoprotein lipase in human adipose tissue." *Journal of Lipid Research* (1992) 33: 89–95.

Westphal, S. A., M. C. Gannon, and F. Q. Nutrall. "Metabolic response to glucose ingested with various amounts of protein." *American Journal of Clinical Nutrition* (1990) 62: 267–272.

Yost, T. J., and R. H. Eckel. "Fat calories may be preferentially stored in reduced-obese women: A permissive pathway for resumption of the obese state." *Journal of Clinical Endocrinology* (1988) 67: 259–264.

CHAPTER 8: YOUR DIETARY ROAD MAP TO THE ZONE

Books
Eades, M. *Thin So Fast.* New York: Warner Books, 1989.

Articles
Baile, C. A., C. L. McLaughlin, and M. A. Della-Fera. "Role of cholecysotokinin and opiod peptides in control of food intake." *Physiology Review* (1986) 66: 172–234.

Del Valle, J., and T. Yamada. "The gut as an endocrine organ." *Annual Review of Medicine* (1990) 41: 447–455.

Friedman, J. E., and P. W. R. Lemon. "Effect of chronic endurance exercise on retention of dietary protein." *International Journal of Sports Medicine* (1989) 10: 118–123.

Gibbs, J., R. D. Young, and G. P. Smith. "Cholecystokinin decreases food intake in rats." *Journal of Comparative Physiology and Psychology* (1973) 84: 488–495.

Gontzea, I., P. Sutzesau, and S. Dumitrache. "The influence of adaptation to physical effort on nitrogen balance in man." *Nutrition Report International* (1975) 11: 231–236.

————. "Influence of muscular activity on nitrogen balance and on the need of man for proteins." *Nutrition Report International* (1974) 10: 35–39.

Jenkins, D. J. A., T. M. S. Wolever, S. Vukson, F. Brighenti, S. C. Cunnane, A. V. Rao, A. L. Jenkins, G. Buckley, and W. Singer. "Nibbling versus gorging: Metabolic advantages of increased meal frequency." *New England Journal of Medicine* (1989) 321: 929–934.

Meredith, C. N., M. J. Zackin, W. R. Frontera, and W. J. Evans. "Dietary protein requirements and body protein metabolism in endurance-training men." *Journal of Applied Physiology* (1989) 6: 2850–2856.

Schwartz, M. W., D. P. Figlewicz, D. G. Baskin, S. C. Woods, and D. Porte. "Insulin in the brain: a hormonal regulation of energy balance." *Endocrine Review* (1992) 43: 387–414.

Tarnopolsky, M. A., J. D. MacDougall, and S. A. Atkinson. "Influence of protein intake and training status on nitrogen balance and lean body mass." *Journal of Applied Physiology* (1988) 64: 187–193.

Welch, I. M. L., C. Bruce, S. E. Hill, and N. W. Reed. "Duodenal and ileal lipid suppresses post-prandial blood glucose and insulin responses in men: Possible implication for dietary management of diabetes mellitus." *Clinical Science* (1987) 72: 209–216.

Wolever, T. M. S., D. J. A. Jenkins, G. R. Collier, R. Lee, G. S. Wong, and R. G. Josse. "Metabolic response to test meals containing different carbohydrate foods: Relationship between rate of digestion and plasma insulin response." *Nutrition Research* (1988) 8: 573–581.

Wolever, T. M. S., D. J. A. Jenkins, A. C. Jenkins, and R. G. Josse. "The glycemic index: methodology and clinical implication." *American Journal of Clinical Nutrition* (1991) 54: 846–854.

CHAPTER 9: EVOLUTION AND THE ZONE

Books

Crawford, M., and D. Marsh. *The Driving Force: Food, Evolution and the Future.* New York: Harper & Row, 1989.

Eaton, S. B., M. Shostalle, and M. Konner. *The Paleolithic Prescription.* New York: Harper & Row, 1988.

Hayflick, L. *How and Why We Age.* New York: Ballantine, 1994.

Articles

Aiello, L. C., and P. Wheeler. "The expensive-tissue hypothesis." *Current Anthropology* (1995) 36: 199–221.

Eaton, S. B., "Humans, lipids and evolution." *Lipids* (1992) 27: 814–820.

Eaton, S. B., and M. J. Konner. "Paleolithic nutrition." *New England Journal of Medicine* (1985) 312: 283–289.

Hollenbeck, C., and G. M. Reaven. "Variations in insulin-stimulated glucose uptake in healthy individuals with normal glucose tolerance." *Journal of Clinical Endocrinology and Metabolism* (1987) 64: 1169–1173.

CHAPTER 10: VITAMINS, MINERALS, AND THE ZONE

Articles

Alpha Tocopherol, Beta Carotene, Cancer Prevention Study Group. "The effect of vitamin E and beta carotene on incidences of lung cancer and other cancers in male smokers." *New England Journal of Medicine* (1994) 330: 1029–1035.

Block, G., B. Patterson, and A. Safar. "Fruit, vegetables and cancer prevention." *Nutrition and Cancer* (1992) 18: 1–29.

Blot, W. J., J. Y. Li, P. R. Taylor, W. Gauo, S. M. Damsey, G. Q. Wang, C. S. Yang, S. F. Zheng, M. Gail, and G. Y. Li. "Nutritional intervention trials in Linxion, China." *Journal of Natural Cancer Research* (1993) 85: 1483–1492.

Colditz, G. A., L. G. Branch, R. J. Lipnick, W. C. Willett, B. Rosner, B. M. Posner, and C. H. Hennekens. "Increased green and leafy vegetable intake and lowered cancer deaths in an elderly population." *American Journal of Clinical Nutrition* (1985) 41: 32–36.

Polyp Prevention Group. "A clinical trial of antioxident vitamins to prevent colorectal ademona." *New England Journal of Medicine* (1994) 331: 141–147.

Rimm, E. B., M. J. Stampfer, A. Ascherio, E. Giovannucci, G. A. Colditz, and W. C. Willett. "Vitamin E consumption and risk of coronary heart disease in men." *New England Journal of Medicine* (1993) 328: 1450–1456.

Shekelle, R. B., M. Lepper, and S. Liu. "Dietary vitamin A and risk of cancer in the Western Electric Study." *Lancet* (1981) 2: 1185–1190.

Stampfer, M. J., C. H. Hennekens, J. E. Mason, G. A. Colditz, B. Rosner, and W. C. Willett. "Vitamin E consumption and risk of coronary disease in women." *New England Journal of Medicine* (1993) 32: 1444–1449.

Steinmetz, K. A., and J. C. Potter. "Vegetables, fruit and cancer." *Cancer Causes Control* (1991) 325: 325–357.

Ziegler, R. G., A. F. Subar, D. E. Craft, G. Ursin, B. H. Patterson, and B. T. Graubard. "Does beta carotene explain why reduced cancer risk is associated with vegetable and fruit intake?" *Cancer Research* (1992) 52: 2060s–2066s.

CHAPTER 11: ASPIRIN: THE WONDER DRUG

Books

Castleman, M. *An Aspirin a Day*. New York: Hyperion, 1993.

Herman, A. G., P. M. Venhoutte, H. Denolin, and A. Gooseen, eds. *Cardiovascular Pharmacology of Prostaglandins*. New York: Raven Press, 1992.

Mann, C. C., and M. L. Plummer. *The Aspirin Wars*. New York: Alfred Knopf, 1991.

Ninneman, J. L. *Prostaglandins, Leukotrienes, and the Immune Response*. New York: Cambridge University Press, 1988.

Articles

Benigni, A., G. Gregorini, T. Frusca, C. Chiabrando, S. Ballerini, A. Volcamonico, S. Orisho, A. Piccelli, V. Pincroli, R. Ianelli, A. Gastaldi, and G. Remuzzi. "Effect of low dose aspirin on fetal and maternal generating thromboxane by platelets in women at risk for pregnancy-induced hypertension." *New England Journal of Medicine* (1989) 321: 357–362.

Brunda, M. J., R. B. Haberman, and H. T. Holden. "Inhibition of natural killer cell activity by prostaglandin." *Journal of Immunology* (1980) 124: 2682–2687.

Burch, J. W., N. Stanford, and P. W. Majerus. "Inhibition of platelet prostaglandin synthesis by oral aspirin." *Journal of Clinical Investigation* (1979) 62: 314–319.

Coceani, F., I. Bishai, N. Hynes, J. Lees, and S. Sirko. "Prostaglandin E$_2$ as central messenger of fevers," in *New Trends in Lipid Mediators Research*, edited by P. Brogeret and L. Robinson. Basel, Switzerland: S. Krager, 1989, pp. 183–186.

Collins, P. W. "Misoprostol: Discovery, development and chemical applications." *Medical Research Review* (1990) 10: 149–172.

Craven, L. L. "Prevention of coronary and cerebral thrombosis." *Mississippi Valley Medical Journal* (1956) 78: 213–218.

Dutch T.I.A. Trial Study Group. "A comparison of two doses of aspirin (30 mg and 283 mg a day) in patients after a transient ischemic attack or minor stroke." *New England Journal of Medicine* (1991) 325: 1261–1266.

Ferreria, S. H., S. Moncada, and J. R. Vane. "Indomethacin and aspirin abolish prostaglandin release from the spleen." *Nature (London) New Biology* (1971) 231: 237–239.

Hamberg, M., J. Svensson, and B. Samuelsson. "Thromboxanes: a new group of biologically active compounds derived from prostaglandin and peroxides." *Proceedings of the National Academy of Science USA* (1975) 72: 2994–2998.

Hawthorne, A. B., Y. R. Mahida, A. T. Cole, and C. J. Hawkey. "Aspirin-induced gastric muscosal damage." *British Journal of Clinical Pharmacology* (1991) 32: 77–83.

Imperiate, T. F., and A. Stollenwerk-Petrulles. "A meta analysis of low-dose aspirin for preventing of pregnancy-induced hypertensive disease." *Journal of the American Medical Association* (1991) 266: 260–264.

Lewis, D. H., J. W. Davis, D. G. Archibald, W. E. Steinte, T. C. Smitherman, J. E. Doherty, H. W. Schnaper, M. M. LeWinter, E. Linares, J. M. Pouget, S. C. Sabharwal, E. Chandler, and H. DeMotis. "Protective effects of aspirin against acute myocardial infarction and death in men with unstable angina." *New England Journal of Medicine* (1983) 309: 396–403.

Paganini-Hill, A., A. Chad, R. K. Ross, and B. E. Henderson. "Aspirin use and chronic diseases." *British Medical Journal* (1989) 299: 1247–1250.

Roth, G. J., N. Stanford, and P. W. Majerus. "Acetylation of prostaglandin synthesase by aspirin." *Proceedings of the National Academy of Science* (1975) 72: 3073–3076.

Roth, G. J., and P. W. Majerus. "The mechanism of the effect of aspirin on human platelets." *Journal of Clinical Investigation* (1975) 50: 624–632.

Roth, G. J., and C. J. Siok. "Acetylation of the NH2-terminal series of prostaglandin synthesase by aspirin." *Journal of Biology and Chemistry* (1975) 253: 3782–3784.

SALT Collaborative Group. "Swedish aspirin low-dose trial (SALT) of 75 mg aspirin as secondary prophylaxis after cerebrovascular schemic agents." *Lancet* (1991) 338: 1345–1349.

Steering Committee of the Physician Health Study Research Group. "Preliminary report findings from the aspirin component of the ongoing physician health study." *New England Journal of Medicine* (1988) 320: 262–264.

Szczeklik, A. "Aspirin induced asthma." *Internal Archives Allergy Applied Immunology* (1989) 90: 70–75.

Taiwo, Y. O., and J. D. Levine. "Prostaglandins inhibit endogenous pain control mechanism by blocking transmission at spinal noradrengenic synapses." *Journal of Neuroscience* (1988) 8: 1346–1349.

Thun, M. J., M. M. Namboodiri, and C. W. Heath. "Aspirin use and reduced risk of fatal colon cancer." *New England Journal of Medicine* (1991) 325: 1593–1596.

Uda, R., S. Horiguchi, S. Ito, M. Hydro, and O. Hayaishi. "Nociceptive effects induced by intrathecal administration of prostaglandins D_2, E_2, or F_2 alpha in conscious mice." *Brain Research* (1990) 510: 26–32.

Vane, J. R. "Inhibition of prostaglandin synthesis as a mechanism of action of aspirinlike drugs." *Nature (London) New Biology* (1971) 231: 232–235.

Weiss, J. H. "Aspirin: A dangerous drug?" *Journal of the American Medical Association* (1974) 229: 1221–1222.

Williams, W. R. "Aspirin-sensitive asthma." *Internal Archives Allergy and Applied Immunology* (1991) 95: 303–308.

CHAPTER 12: THE WONDER HORMONES: EICOSANOIDS—THE LONG COURSE

Books

Herman, A. G., P. M. Van houtle, H. Denolin, and A. Goosen, eds. *Cardiovascular Pharmacology of the Prostaglandins.* New York: Raven Press, 1982.

Jensen, R. G. *The Lipids of Human Milk.* Boca Raton, FL: CRC Press, 1989.

Lands, W. E. M. *Fish and Human Health.* New York: Academic Press, 1986.

Ninneman, J. L. *Prostaglandins, Leukotrienes, and the Immune Response.* New York: Cambridge University Press, 1988.

Schor, K., and H. Sinziner, eds. *Prostaglandins in Clinical Research.* New York: Wiley-Liss, 1989.

Sinclair, A., and R. Gibson. *Essential Fatty Acids and Eicosanoids.* Champaign, IL: American Oil and Chemical Society Press, 1992.

Sinzinger, H., and W. Rogatti, eds. *Prostaglandin E_1 in Atherosclerosis.* New York: Springer-Verlag, 1986.

Watkins, W. D., M. B. Petersen, and J. R. Fletcher, eds. *Prostaglandins in Clinical Practice.* New York: Raven Press, 1989.

Willis, A. L. *Handbook of Eicosanoids, Prostaglandins and Related Lipids.* Boca Raton, FL: CRC Press, 1987.

Articles

Adam, O. "Polyenoic fatty acid metabolism and effects on prostaglandin biosynthesis in adults and aged persons," in *Polyunsaturated Fatty Acids and Eicosanoids*. Champaign, IL: American Oil and Chemical Society Press, 1987, pp. 213–219.

Addison, R. F., and R. G. Ackman. "Removal of organic chlorine pesticides and polychlorinated biphenyls from marine oils during refining and hydrogenation for edible use." *Journal of the American Oil and Chemical Society* (1974) 51: 192–194.

Addison, R. F., M. E. Zinck, R. G. Ackman, and J. C. Sipos. "Behavior of DDT, polychlorinated bybeniyls (PCB's) and dieldrin at various stages of refining of marine oils for edible use." *Journal of the American Oil and Chemical Society* (1978) 55: 391–394.

Ayala, S., G. Gasper, R. R. Brenner, R. Peluffo, and W. J. Kunau. "Fate of linoleic, arachidonic and docosatetraonoic acids in rat testicles." *Journal of Lipid Research* (1973) 14: 296–305.

Blond, J. P., and P. Lemarchel. "A study on the effect of alpha linolenic acid on the desaturation of dihomo gamma linolenic acid using rat liver homogenates." *Reproductive Nutrition Development* (1984) 24: 1–10.

Bourre, J. M., M. Piciotti, and O. Dumont. "Delta 6 desaturase in brain and liver during development and aging." *Lipids* (1990) 25: 354–356.

Brenner, R. R. "Nutrition and hormonal factors influencing desaturation of essential fatty acids." *Progressive Lipid Research* (1982) 20: 41–48.

Chapkin, R. S., S. D. Somer, and K. L. Erickson. "Dietary manipulation of macrophage phospholipid classes: Selective increase of dihomogamma linoleic acid." *Lipids* (1988) 23: 776–770.

Cleland, L. G., M. J. Jones, M. A. Neuman, M. D'Angel, and R. A. Gibson. "Linoleate inhibits EPA incorporation from dietary fish oil supplements in human subjects." *American Journal of Clinical Nutrition* (1992) 55: 395–399.

Collins, P. W. "Misoprostol: Discovery, development and chemical applications." *Medical Research Review* (1990) 10: 149–172.

Earle, C. M., E. J. Kenough, Z. S. Wisniewski, A. G. S. Tulloch, D. J. Lord, G. R. Walters, and C. Glatthear. "Prostaglandin E_1 therapy for impotence, comparison with papaverine." *Journal of Urology* (1990) 143: 57–79.

Gann, P. H. "Prospective study of plasma fatty acids and risk of prostate cancer." *Journal of the National Cancer Institute* (1994) 86: 281–286.

Garcia, P. T., and R. T. Holman. "Competitive inhibitions in the metabolism of polyunsaturated fatty acids studied via the composition of the phospholipids, triglycerides and cholesterol esters of rat tissues." *Journal of the American Oil and Chemical Society* (1965) 42: 1137–1141.

Gauglitz, E. J., and E. H. Greegan. "Adsorptive bleaching and molecular distillation of menhaden oil." *Journal of the American Oil and Chemical Society* (1965) 42: 561–563.

Gibson, R. A., and G. M. Kneebone. "Fatty acid composition of human colostrum and mature human milk." *American Journal of Clinical Nutrition* (1981) 34: 252–256.

Giovannucci, E., E. B. Rimm, G. A. Colditz, M. J. Stampfer, A. Ascherio, C. C. Chute, and W. C. Willett. "Prospective study of dietary fat and risk of prostate cancer." *Journal of the National Cancer Institute* (1993) 85: 1571–1579.

Giovannucci, E., E. B. Rimm, M. J. Stampfer, G. A. Colditz, A. Ascherio, and W. C. Wiillett. "Intake of fat, meat, and fiber in relation to risk of colon cancer in men." *Cancer Research* (1994) 54: 2390–2397.

Hill, E. G., S. B. Johnson, L. D. Lawson, M. M. Mahfouz, and R. T. Holman. "Perturbation of the metabolism of essential fatty acids by dietary partially hydrogenated vegetable oil." *Proceedings of the National Academy of Science USA* (1982) 79: 953–957.

Horrobin, D. F. "Loss of delta 6 desatures activity as a key factor in aging." *Medical Hypothesis* (1981) 7: 1211–1220.

Kirtland, S. J. "Prostaglandin E_1: A review." *Prostaglandins, Leukotrienes and Essential Fatty Acids* (1988) 32: 165–174.

Koosis, V., and J. Sondergaard. "PGE_1 in normal skin: Methodological evaluation, topographical distribution and data related to sex and age." *Archives of Dermatology Research* (1983) 275: 9–13.

Mensink, R. P., and M. B. Katan. "Effect of dietary trans–fatty acids on high-density and low-density lipoprotein levels in healthy subjects." *New England Journal of Medicine* (1990) 323: 439–445.

Nassar, B. A., Y. S. Huang, M. S. Manku, U. M. Das, N. Morse, and

D. F. Horrobin. "The influence of dietary manipulation with n-3 and n-6 fatty acids on liver and plasma phospholipids fatty acids in rats." *Lipids* (1986) 21: 652–656.

Phinney, S. "Potential risk of prolonged gamma-linolenic acid use." *Annual Internal Medicine* (1994) 120: 692.

Schofield, J. G. "Prostaglandin E_1 and the release of growth hormone in vitro." *Nature* (1970) 228: 179.

See, J., W. Shell, O. Matthews, C. Canizales, M. Vargos, J. Giddings, and J. Cerrone. "Prostaglandin E_1 infusion after angioplasty in humans inhibits abrupt occlusion and early restenosis." *Advances in Prostoglandin Thromboxane, and Leukotriene Research* (1987) 17: 266–270.

Stone, K. J., A. L. Willis, M. Hurt, S. J. Kirtland, P. B. A. Kernoff, and G. F. McNichol. "The metabolism of dihomo gamma linolenic acid in man." *Lipids* (1979) 14: 174–180.

Williams, L. L., D. M. Doody, and L. A. Horrocks. "Serum fatty acid proportions are altered during the year following acute Epstein-Barr virus infection." *Lipids* (1988) 23: 981–988.

CHAPTER 13: THE ZONE AND YOUR HEART

Books

Bernstein, R. K. *Diabetes Type II.* New York: Prentice-Hall Press, 1990.

Lands, W. E. M. *Fish and Human Health.* New York: Academic Press, 1986.

Moore, T. J. *Heart Failure.* New York: Random House, 1989.

———. *Lifespan.* New York: Simon and Schuster, 1993.

Sinzinger, H., and W. Rogatti, eds. *Prostaglandin E_1 in Atherosclerosis.* New York: Spinger-Verlag, 1986.

Articles

Baba, T., and S. Neugebauer. "The link between insulin resistance and hypertension: effects of antihypertensive and antihyperlipidaemic drugs on insulin sensitivity." *Drugs* (1994) 47: 383–404.

Black, H. R. "The coronary artery disease paradox: The role of hype-

rinsulinemia and insulin resistance and implications for therapy." *Journal of Cardiovascular Pharmacology* (1990) 15: 26S–38S.

Blankenhorn, D. H., S. P. Azen, D. M. Kramsch, M. J. Mack, L.
Cashlin-Hemphill, H. N. Hodis, L. W. V. DeBoer, R. P.
Mahrer, M. J. Masteller, L. I. Vailas, P. Alaupovic, L. J. Hirsch,
and MARS Research Group. "Coronary angiographic changes
with lovastatin therapy: The monitored atherosclerotic regression study (MARS)." *Annual Internal Medicine* (1993) 119: 969–
976.

Blankenhorn, D. H., S. A. Nessim, R. L. Johnson, M. E. Sanmarco,
S. P. Azen, and L. Cashlin-Hamphill. "Beneficial effects of combined colestipol-niacin therapy in coronary atherosclerosis and
coronary venous bypass grafts." *Journal of the American Medical
Association* (1987) 257: 3233–3240.

Brenner, R. R. "Nutritional and hormonal factors influencing
desaturation of essential fatty acids." *Progressive Lipid Research*
(1982) 20: 41–47.

Burnand, B., and A. R. Feinstein. "The role of diagnostic inconsistency in changing rates of occurrence for coronary heart disease."
Journal of Clinical Epidemiology (1992) 45: 929–940.

Chen, Y. D., A. M. Coulston, Z. Ming-Yue, C. B. Hollenbeck, and
G. M. Reaven. "Why do low-fat high-carbohydrate diets accen-
tuate postprandial lipemia in patients with NIDDM?" *Diabetes
Care* (1995) 18: 10–16.

Committee of Principal Investigators. "A co-operative trial in primary prevention of ischemic heart disease using clofibrate."
British Heart Journal (1978) 40: 1069–1118.

Dayton, S., and M. L. Pearce. "Prevention of coronary heart disease
and other complications of arteriosclerosis by modified diet."
American Journal of Medicine (1969) 46: 751–762.

Dehmer, G. J., J. J. Popma, E. K. van den Ber, E. J. Eichorn, J. B.
Prewitt, W. B. Campbell, L. Jennings, J. T. Willerson, and J. M.
Schmitz. "Reduction in the rate of early restenosis after coro-
nary angioplasty by a diet supplemented with n-3 fatty acids."
New England Journal of Medicine (1988) 319: 733–740.

Donahue, R. R., R. D. Abbott, E. Bloom, D. M. Reed, and K. Yano.
"Central obesity and coronary heart disease in men." *Lancet*
(1987) 1: 820–823.

Ducimetière, P., E. Eschwege, G. Papoz, J. L. Richard, J. R. Claude, and G. Rosselin. "Relationship of plasma insulin to the incidence of myocardial infarction and coronary heart disease mortality in a middle-aged population." *Diabetologia* (1980) 19: 205–210.

Ducimetrière, P., J. L. Richard, and I. Cambrien. "The pattern of subcutaneous fat distribution in middle-aged men and risk of coronary heart disease." *International Journal of Obesity* (1986) 10: 229–240.

Eschwege, E., J. L. Richard, N. Thibult, P. Ducimetière, J. M. Warsnot, J. R. Claude, and G. E. Rosselin. "Coronary heart disease mortality in relation to diabetes, blood glucose, and plasma insulin levels." *Hormone Metabolism Research Supplement* (1985) 15: 41–46.

Facchini, F. S., C. B. Hollenbeck, J. Jeppeson, Y. D. Chen, and G. M. Reaven. "Insulin resistance and cigarette smoking." *Lancet* (1992) 339: 1128–1130.

Farquhar, J. W., A. Frank, R. C. Gross, and G. M. Reaven. "Glucose, insulin, and triglyceride responses to high and low carbohydrate diets in man." *Journal of Clinical Investigation* (1966) 45: 1648–1656.

Ferrannini, E., G. Buzzigoli, R. Bonadonna, M. A. Giorico, M. Oleggini, L. Grazideli, R. Pedrinelli, L. Brand, and S. Beviacqua. "Insulin resistance in essential hypertension." *New England Journal of Medicine* (1987) 317: 350–357.

Foster, D. "Insulin resistance—A secret killer?" *New England Journal of Medicine* (1989) 320: 733–734.

Frantz, I. D., E. A. Dawson, P. L. Ashman, L. C. Gatewood, G. E. Barsch, K. Kuba, and E. R. Brewer. "Test of effect of lipid lowering by diet on cardiovascular risk: The Minnesota coronary survey." *Arteriosclerosis* (1989) 9: 129–135.

Frick, H. M., O. Elo, K. Haapa, O. P. Keinonem, P. Heinsalmi, P. Halo, J. K. Huttunen, P. Kaitaniemi, P. Koskinen, V. Manninen, H. Maenapaa, M. Malkonen, M. Manttari, S. Norola, A. Pasternack, J. Pikkarinen, M. Romo, P. Sjoblom, and E. A. Mikkla. "Helsinki Heart Study: Primary prevention trial with gemfibrozil in middle-aged men with hyperlipidemia." *New England Journal of Medicine* (1987) 317: 1237–1245.

Garg, A., J. P. Bantle, R. R. Henry, A. M. Coulston, K. A. Griven, S. K. Raatz, L. Brinkley, I. Chen, S. M. Grundy, B. A. Huet, and G. M. Reaven. "Effects of varying carbohydrate content of diet in patients with non-insulin-dependent diabetes mellitus." *Journal of the American Medical Association* (1994) 271: 1421–1428.

Garg, A., S. M. Grudy, and R. H. Unger. "Comparison of effects of high and low carbohydrate diets on plasma lipoproteins and insulin sensitivity in patients with mild NIDDM." *Diabetes* (1992) 41: 1278–1285.

Gaziano, J. M., J. E. Burning, J. L. Breslow, S. Z. Goldhaber, B. Rosner, M. van Denburgh, W. C. Willett, and C. H. Hennekens. "Moderate alcohol intake, increased levels of high-density lipoproteins and its subfractions, and decreased risk of myocardial infarctions." *New England Journal of Medicine* (1993) 329: 1829–1834.

Gertler, M. H., E. Leetma, E. Saluste, J. L. Rosenberger, and R. G. Guthrie. "Ischemic heart disease, insulin, carbohydrate and lipid inter-relationship." *Circulation* (1972) 46: 103–111.

Ginsberg, H., J. M. Olefsky, G. Kimmerling, P. Crapo, and G. M. Reaven. "Induction of hypertriglyceridemia by a low-fat diet." *Journal of Clinical Endocrinology* (1976) 42: 729–735.

Grunze, M., and B. Deuticke. "Changes of membrane permeability due to extensive cholesterol depletion in mammalian erthrocytes." *Biochemical Biophysics Acta* (1974) 356: 125–130.

Gruss, J. D. "Experience with PGE_1 in patients with phlemgasia coerulea dolens and ergothism," in *Prostaglandin E_1 in Atherosclerosis*, edited by H. Sinzinger and W. Rogatti. New York: Spinger-Verlag, 1986, pp. 97–105.

Hach, W., B. W. Zanke, G. Sauerwein, and Y. Ozen. "Treatment of Stage IIb peripheral arterial occlusive disease with short-term intra-arterial infusion of prostaglandin E_1," in *Prostaglandin E_1 in Atherosclerosis*, edited by H. Sinzinger and W. Rogatti. New York: Spinger-Verlag, 1986, pp. 66–74.

Hjermann, I., I. Home, K. Velve-Byre, and P. Leren. "Effect of diet and smoking intervention on incidence of coronary heart disease." *Lancet* (1981) 2: 1303–1310.

Hollenbeck, C., and G. M. Reaven. "Variation of insulin stimulated glucose uptake in healthy individuals with normal glucose tolerance." *Journal of Clinical Endocrinology and Metabolism* (1987) 64: 1169–1173.

Hrboticky, N., B. Tang, B. Zimmer, I. Lux, and P. C. Weber. "Lovastatin increases arachidonic acid levels and stimulates thromboxane synthesis in human liver and monocytic cell lines." *Journal of Clinical Investigation* (1994) 93: 195–203.

Jones, P. M., and S. J. Persaud. "Arachidonic acid as a second messenger in glucose-induced insulin secretion from pancreatic beta cells." *Journal of Endocrinology* (1993) 137: 7–14.

Kannel, W. B., J. T. Doyle, A. M. Ostfield, C. D. Jenkins, L. Kuller, R. N. Podell, and J. Stemler. "Optimal resources for primary prevention of atherosclerotic diseases." *Circulation* (1984) 70: 157A–205A.

Kaplan, N. "The deadly quartet: Upper body obesity, glucose intolerance, hypertriglyceridemia, and hypertension." *Archives of Internal Medicine* (1989) 149: 1514–1520.

Knapp, H. R., I. A. G. Reilly, P. Alessandrini, and G. A. FitzGerald. "In vivo indexes of platelet and vascular function during fish-oil administration in patients with atherosclerosis." *New England Journal of Medicine* (1986) 314: 937–942.

Kromhout, D., E. B. Bosscheter, and C. L. Coulander. "The inverse relationship between fish consumption and 20-year mortality from coronary heart disease." *New England Journal of Medicine* (1985) 312: 1205–1209.

Krone, W., A. Klass, H. Nagele, B. Behnke, and H. Greten. "Effects of prostaglandin E_1 on low-density lipoprotein receptor activity and cholesterol synthesis in freshly isolated human mononuclear leukocytes," in *Prostaglandin E_1 in Atherosclerosis*, edited by W. Rogatti and H. Sinzinger. New York: Spinger-Verlag, 1986, pp. 32–38.

Krumholz, H. M., T. E. Seeman, S. S. Merrill, C. F. Mendes de Leon, V. Vaccarino, D. I. Silverman, R. Tsukahara, A. M. Ostfield, and L. F. Berkman. "Lack of association between cholesterol and coronary heart disease mortality and morbidity and all-cause mortality in persons older than 70 years." *Journal of the American Medical Association* (1994) 272: 1335–1340.

Kuczmarshi, R. J., K. M. Flegal, S. M. Campbell, and C. L. Johnson. "Increasing relevance of overweight among U.S. adults." *Journal of the American Medical Association* (1994) 272: 205–211.

Lakshmanan, M. R., C. M. Nepokroeff, G. C. Ness, R. E. Dugan, and J. W. Porter. "Stimulation by insulin of rat liver beta hydroxy methyl HMGCoA and cholesterol synthesizing activities." *Biochemical and Biophysics Research Committee* (1973) 50: 704–710.

Larsson, B., K. Svarsudd, L. Welin, L. Wilhelmssen, P. Bjorntorp, and G. Tilbin. "Abdominal adipose tissue distribution, obesity and risk of cardiovascular disease and death." *British Medical Journal* (1984) 288: 1401–1404.

Laws, A., A. C. King, W. L. Haskell, and G. M. Reaven. "Relation of fasting plasma insulin concentrations to high density lipoprotein cholesterol and triglyceride concentrations in man." *Arteriosclerosis and Thrombosis* (1991) 11: 1636–1642.

Lewis, D. H., J. W. Davis, D. G. Archibald, W. E. Steinte, T. C. Smitherman, J. E. Doherty, H. W. Schnaper, M. M. LeWinter, E. Linares, J. M. Pouget, S. C. Sabharwal, E. Chandler, and H. DeMotis. "Protective effects of aspirin against acute myocardial infarction and death in men with unstable angina." *New England Journal of Medicine* (1983) 309: 396–403.

MAAS Investigators. "Effect of simvastatin on coronary atheroma: The multicentre anti-atheroma study (MAAS)." *Lancet* (1994) 344: 633–638.

McCormick, J., and P. Skrabanek. "Coronary heart disease is not preventable by population interventions." *Lancet* (1988) 2: 839–841.

Medical Research Council Working Party. "MRC trial of treatment of mild hypertension." *British Medical Journal* (1985) 291: 97–104.

Modan, M., J. Or, A. Karasik, Y. Drory, Z. Fuchs, A. Lusky, and A. Cherit. "Hyperinsulinemia, sex, and risk of athersclerotic cardiovascular disease." *Circulation* (1991) 84: 1165–1175.

Morgan, W. A., P. Paskin, and J. Rosenstock. "A comparison of fish oil or corn oil supplements in hyperlipidemic subjects with NIDDM." *Diabetes Care* (1995) 18: 83–86.

Morrow, J. D., B. Frei, A. W. Longmire, J. M. Gaziano, S. M. Lynch, Y. Shyr, W. E. Strauss, J. A. Oates, and L. J. Roberts. "Increase in circulating products of lipid peroxidation (F2-isoprosotanes) in smokers." *New England Journal of Medicine* (1995) 332: 1198–1203.

Muldoon, M. F., S. B. Manrick, and K. A. Matthews. "Lowering cholesterol concentrations and mortality: a quantitative review of primary prevention trials." *British Medical Journal* (1990) 301: 309–314.

Multiple Risk Factor Intervention Trial Research Group. "Multiple risk factor intervention trial." *Journal of the American Medical Association* (1982) 248: 1465–1477.

Nestler, J. E., N. A. Beer, D. J. Jakubowicz, C. Colombo, and R. M. Beer. "Effects of insulin reduction with benfluorex on serum dehydroepiandrosterone (DHEA), DHEA sulfate, and blood pressure in hypertensive middle-aged and elderly men." *Journal of Clinical Endocrinology and Metabolism* (1995) 80: 700–706.

Oates, J. A., G. A. FitzGerald, R. A. Branch, E. K. Jackson, H. P. Knapp, and L. J. Roberts. "Clinical implications of prostaglandin and thromboxane A_2 formation." *New England Journal of Medicine* (1988) 319: 689–698, 761–767.

Ornish, D. S. E. Brown, L. W. Scherwitz, J. H. Billings, R. L. Kirkeeide, R. J. Brand, and K. L. Gould. "Can lifestyle changes reverse coronary heart disease?" *Lancet* (1990) 336: 129–133.

Parillo, M., A. A. Rivellese, A. V. Ciardullo, B. Capaldo, A. Giacco, S. Genovese, and G. Riccardi. "A high-monounsaturated-fat/low-carbohydrate diet improves peripheral insulin sensitivity in non-insulin dependent diabetic patients." *Metabolism* (1992) 41: 1373–1378.

Pelikanov, T., M. Kohout, J. Base, Z. Steka, J. Dovar, L. D'Azdova, and J. Valek. "Effect of acute hyperinsulinemia on fatty acid composition of serum lipids in non-insulin dependent diabetics and healthy men." *Clinica Chemica Acta* (1991) 203: 329–338.

Peris, A. N., M. S. Slothmann, R. G. Hoffman, M. J. Hennes, C. R. Wilson, A. B. Gustafson, and A. H. Kissbah. "Adiposity, fat distribution and cardiovascular risk." *Annual Internal Medicine* (1989) 110: 867–872.

Pyorala, K., E. Savolainen, S. Kaukula, and J. Haapakowski. "Plasma insulin as coronary heart disease risk factor." *Academy of Medicine Scandinavia* (1985) 701: 38–52.

Reaven, G. M. "The role of insulin resistance and hyperinsulinemia in coronary heart disease." *Metabolism* (1992) 41: 16–19.

———. "Role of insulin resistance in human disease." *Diabetes* (1989) 37: 1595–1607.

———. "Syndrome X: 6 years later." *Journal of Internal Medicine Supplement* (1994) 736: 13–22.

Reaven, G. M., and B. Hoffman. "Abnormalities of carbohydrate metabolism may play a role in the etiology and clinical course of hypertension." *Trends in Pharmacological Science* (1988) 9: 78–79.

Renaud, S., and M. de Lorgeril. "Wine alcohol, platelets and the French paradox for coronary heart disease." *Lancet* (1992) 339: 1523–1526.

Rodwell, V. W., J. L. Nordstrom, and J. J. Mitschelen. "Regulation of HMG-CoA reductase." *Advances in Lipid Research* (1976) 14: 1–76.

Ross, R. "The pathogenesis of atherosclerosis." *New England Journal of Medicine* (1986) 314: 488–500.

Ruderman, N., and C. Haudenschild. "Diabetes as an atherogenic factor." *Progress in Cardiovascular Diseases* (1984) 26: 373–412.

Sacca, L., G. Perez, F. Pengo, I. Pascucci, and M. Conorelli. "Reduction of circulating insulin levels during the infusion of different prostaglandins in the rat." *Acta Endocrinology* (1975) 79: 266–274.

Scandinavian Simvastatin Survival Study Group. "Randomised trial of cholesterol lowering in 4444 patients with coronary heart disease: the Scandinavian simvastatin survival study (4S)." *Lancet* (1994) 344: 1383–1389.

Schwartz, L. C. J., A. J. Valente, E. A. Sprague, J. L. Kelley, A. J. Cayatte, and M. M. Rozek. "Pathogenesis of the atherosclerotic lesion." *Diabetes Care* (1992) 15: 1156–1167.

Shepard, J., S. M. Cobbe, I. Ford, C. G. Isles, A. R. Lorimer, P. W. MacFarlane, J. H. McKillop, and C. J. Packard. "Prevention of coronary heart disease with pravastatin in men with hypercholesterolemia." *New England Journal of Medicine* (1995) 333: 1301–1307.

Sheu, W. H., S. M. Shieh, D. D. Shen, M. M. Fuh, C. Y. Jeng, Y. D. Chen, and G. M. Reaven. "Effect of pravastatin treatment on glucose, insulin, and lipoprotein metabolism in patients with hypercholesterolemia." *American Heart Journal* (1994) 127: 331–336.

Silver, M. J., W. Hock, J. J. Kocsis, C. M. Ingerman, and J. B. Smith. "Arachidonic acid causes sudden death in rabbits." *Science* (1974) 183: 1085–1087.

Sinzinger, H. "Inhibition of mitotic and proliferative activity of smooth muscle cell by prostaglandin E," in *Prostaglandin E_1 in Atherosclerosis*, edited by W. Rogatti and H. Sinzinger. New York: Spinger-Verlag, 1986, pp. 37–48.

Smith, D. L., A. L. Willis, N. Nguyen, D. Conner, S. Zahedi, and J. Fulks. "Eskimo plasma constituents, dihomo gamma linolenic acid, eicosapentaenoic acid and docosahexaenoic acid inhibit the release of atherogenic mitogens." *Lipids* (1989) 24: 70–75.

Stein, P. P., and H. R. Block. "Drug treatment of hypertension in patients with diabetes amellitus." *Diabetes Care* (1991) 14: 425–448.

Stern, M. P., and S. M. Haffner. "Body fat distribution and hyperinsulinemia as risk factors for diabetes and cardiovascular disease." *Arteriosclerosis* (1986) 6: 123–130.

Steering Committee of Physicians Health Study Research Group. "Preliminary Report: Finds for aspirin component of the on-going physician health study." *New England Journal of Medicine* (1988) 320: 262–264.

Stolar, M. "Atherosclerosis in diabetes: The role of hyperinsulinemia." *Metabolism* (1988) 37: 1–9.

Stout, R. "Insulin and atheroma—An update." *Lancet* (1987) 1: 1077–1079.

———. "The relationship of abnormal circulating insulin levels to atherosclerosis." *Atherosclerosis* (1977) 27: 1–13.

Waters, D., L. Higginson, P. Gladstone, B. Kimball, M. LeMay, S. J. Boccuzzi, J. Lesperance, and CCAIT Study Group. "Effects of monotherapy with HMG-CoA reductase inhibitor on progression of atherosclerosis as assessed by serial arteriography: The Canadian coronary atherosclerosis intervention trial (CCAIT)." *Circulation* (1994) 89: 959–968.

Welborn, T. A., and K. Wearne. "Coronary heart disease incidence and cardiovascular mortality in Brusselton with reference to glucose and insulin concentrations." *Diabetes Care* (1979) 2: 154–160.

WHO European Collaborative Group. "European collaborative trial of multifactoral prevention of coronary heart disease: Final report on 6-year results." *Lancet* (1986) 1: 869–872.

———. "Multifactoral trial in the prevention of coronary heart disease: 3. Incidence and mortality results." *European Heart Journal* (1983) 4: 141–147.

Wilhelmsen, L., G. Berglund, and D. Elmfeldt. "The multifactoral primary prevention trial in Göteborg, Sweden." *European Heart Journal* (1981) 7: 279–288.

Zavaroni, I., E. Bonora, M. Pagliara, E. Dall'Aglio, L. Luchetti, G. Buonnanno, P. A. Bonati, M. Bergonzani, L. Bnudi, M. Passeri, and G. M. Reaven. "Risk factors for coronary artery disease in healthy persons with hyperinsulinemia and normal glucose tolerance." *New England Journal of Medicine* (1989) 320: 702–706.

Zavaroni, I., L. Bonini, M. Fantuzi, E. Dall'Aglio, M. Passeri, and G. M. Reaven. "Hyperinsulinemia, obesity, and syndrome X." *Journal of Internal Medicine* (1994) 235: 51–56.

Zimmet, P., and S. Baba. "Central obesity, glucose intolerance and other cardiovascular risk factors." *Diabetes Research for Clinical Procedures* (1990) 16: S167–S171.

CHAPTER 14: CANCER AND THE ZONE

Books

Kushi, M., and A. Kushi. *Macrobiotic Diet.* New York: Japan Publications, 1985.

Ninnemann, J. L. *Prostaglandins, Leukotrienes, and the Immune Response.* New York: Cambridge Press, 1988.

Quillin, P. *Beating Cancer with Nutrition.* Tulsa, OK: Nutrition Times Press, 1994.

Tahler-Dao, H., A. Crastes de Paulet, and R. Paoletti, eds. *Icosanoids and Cancer.* New York: Raven Press, 1984.

Weindruch, R., and R. L. Walford. *The Relationship of Aging and Disease by Dietary Restriction.* Springfield, IL: C. C. Thomas, 1988.

Articles

Bailar, J. C., and E. M. Smith. "Progress against cancer?" *New England Journal of Medicine* (1986) 314: 1226–1232.

Bankhurst, A. D. "Modulation of human natural killer cell activity by prostaglandins." *Journal of Clinical Laboratory Immunology* (1982) 7: 85–91.

Braverman, A. S. "Medical Oncology in the 1990s." *Lancet* (1991) 337: 901–902.

Bruning, P. F., M. G. Bonfrer, P. A. H. van Noord, A. A. M. Hart, M. de Jong-Bakken, and W. J. Nooijen. "Insulin resistance and breast cancer." *International Journal of Cancer* (1992) 52: 511–516.

Chapkin, R. S., S. D. Somers, and K. L. Erickson. "Dietary manipulation of macrophage phospholipid classes." *Lipids* (1988) 23: 766–770.

Enders, S., R. Ghorbani, V. E. Kelly, K. Georgilis, G. Lonneman, J. W. M. van der Meer, J. G. Cannon, T. S. Rogers, M. S. Klempner, P. C. Weber, E. J. Schaefer, S. M. Wolff, and C. A. Dinarello. "The effect of dietary supplementation with n-3 polyunsaturated fatty acids on the synthesis of interleukin-1 and tumor necrosis factor by mononuclear cells." *New England Journal of Medicine* (1989) 320: 265–271.

Folkman, J. "What is the evidence that tumors are angiogenesis dependent?" *Journal of the National Cancer Institute* (1990) 82: 4–6.

Giovannucci, E., E. B. Rimm, G. A. Colditz, M. J. Stampfer, A. Ascherio, C. C. Chute, and W. C. Willett. "A prospective study of dietary fat and risk of prostate cancer." *Journal of the National Cancer Institute* (1993) 85: 1571–1579.

Giovannucci, E., E. B. Rimm, M. J. Stampfer, G. A. Colditz, A. Ascherio, and W. C. Willett. "Intake of fat, meat, and fiber in relation to risk of colon cancer in men." *Cancer Research* (1994) 54: 2390–2397.

Gordon, D., M. A. Bray, and J. Morley. "Control of hymphokine secretion by prostaglandins." *Nature* (1976) 262: 401–402.

Grant, J. P. "Proper use and recognized role of TPN in the cancer patient." *Nutrition* (1990) 6: 6S–7S.

Honn, K. V., K. K. Nelson, C. Renaud, R. Bazaz, C. A. Diglio, and J. Timar. "Fatty acid modulation of tumor cell adhesion to microvessel endothelium and experimental metasis." *Prostaglandins* (1992) 44: 413–429.

Kaye, S. A., A. R. Folsom, J. T. Soler, R. J. Prineas, and J. D. Patten. "Association of body mass and fat distribution in sex hormone concentrations in post menopausal women." *International Journal of Epidemiology* (1991) 20: 151–156.

Leung, K. H., and H. S. Koren. "Regulation of human natural killing: Protective effect of interferon on NK cells and suppression by PGE_2." *Journal of Immunology* (1982) 129: 1742–1747.

Liu, B., L. J. Marnett, A. Chaudhary, C. Ji, I. A. Blair, C. R. Johnson, C. A. Diglio, and K. V. Honn. "Biosynthesis of 12-hydroxy eicosatetraenoic acid by B_{16} amelanotic melanoma cells is a determinant of their metastatic potential." *Laboratory Investigation* (1994) 70: 314–323.

Meydani, S. N. "Modulation of cytokine production by dietary polyunsaturated fatty acids." *Proceedings of the Society for Experimental Biology Medicine* (1992) 200: 189–193.

Murota, S., T. Kanayasu, J. Nakano-Hayashi, and I. Morita. "Involvement of eicosanoids in angiogenesis." *Advanced Prostaglandins, Thromboxanes and Leukotriene Research* (1990) 21: 623–625.

Nasser, B. A., Y. S. Huang, M. S. Manku, U. N. Das, N. Morse, and D. F. Horrobin. "The influence of dietary manipulation with n-3 and n-6 fatty acids on liver and plasma phospholids in rats." *Lipids* (1986) 21: 652–656.

Okusawa, S., J. A. Gelfand, T. Ikejima, R. J. Connolly, and C. A. Dinarello. "Interleukin 1 induces a shock-like state in rabbits. Synergism with tumor necrosis factor and the effect of cyclooxygenase inhibition." *Journal of Clinical Investigation* (1988) 82: 1162–1172.

Rappaport, R. S., and G. R. Dodge. "Prostaglandin E inhibits the production of human interleukin 2." *Journal of Experimental Medicine* (1982) 155: 943–948.

Schapira, D. V., N. B. Kumar, G. H. Lyman, and C. E. Cox. "Abdominal obesity and breast cancer risk." *Annual Internal Medicine* (1990) 112: 182–186.

Schartzken, A., P. Greewold, D. P. Byar, and C. K. Clifford. "The dietary fat–breast cancer hypothesis is alive." *Journal of the American Medical Association* (1989) 261: 3284–3287.

Seller, T. A., L. Kushi, J. D. Potter, S. A. Kaye, C. L. Nelson, P. G. McGovern, and A. R. Folsom. "Effect of family history, body fat distribution, and reproductive factors on the risk of post-menopausal breast cancer." *New England Journal of Medicine* (1992) 326: 1323–1329.

Serhan, C. N. "Lipoxin biosynthesis and its impact in inflammatory and vascular events." *Biochemica Biophysica Acta* (1994) 1212: 1–25.

Temple, N. J., and D. P. Burkitt. "The war on cancer—Failure of therapy and research." *Journal of the Royal Society of Medicine* (1991) 84: 95–98.

Weindruch, R. "Effect of caloric restriction on age-associated cancers." *Experimental Gerontology* (1992) 27: 575–581.

Willett, W. C., D. J. Hunter, M. J. Stampfer, G. Colditz, J. E. Manson, D. Spegelman, B. Rosner, C. H. Hennekens, and F. E. Speizer. "Dietary fat and fiber in relation to risk of breast cancer." *Journal of the American Medical Association* (1992) 268: 2037–2044.

CHAPTER 15: CHRONIC DISEASES AND THE ZONE

Books

Gilman, A. G., T. W. Rall, A. S. Nies, and P. Taylor, eds. *The Pharmacological Basis of Therapeutics.* 8th ed. New York: Pergamon Press, 1990.

Horrobin, D. F., ed. *Omega 6 Essential Fatty Acids.* New York: Wiley-Liss, 1990.

Jefferies, W. M. *Safe Uses of Cortisone.* Springfield, IL: C. C. Thomas, 1981.

Root-Bernstein, R. *Rethinking AIDS.* New York: Free Press, 1993.

Ruzicka, T., ed. *Eicosanoids and the Skin.* Boca Raton, FL: CRC Press, 1990.

Schlemier, R. P., H. N. Claman, and A. Oronsky, eds. *Anti-Inflammatory Steroid Action.* San Diego: Academic Press, 1989.

Articles

Abdulla, Y. H., and K. Hamadah. "Effect of ADP on PGE formation in blood platelets from patients with depression, mania, and schizophrenia." *British Journal of Psychiatry* (1975) 127: 591–595.

Aberg, J. "Prostaglandin production in chronic progressive multiple sclerosis." *Journal of Clinical Laboratory Analysis* (1990) 4: 226–250.

Ascher, M. S., and H. W. Sheppard. "AIDS as immune system activation." *Journal of Acquired Immune Deficiency Syndromes* (1990) 3: 177–191.

Bamford, J. T. M., R. W. Gibson, and C. M. Reiner. "Atopic eczema unresponsive to evening primrose oil." *Journal of the American Academy of Dermatology* (1985) 13: 959–965.

Behan, P. O., W. M. H. Behan, and D. F. Horrobin. "Effect of high doses of essential fatty acids on postviral fatigue syndrome." *Acta Neurology Scandinavia* (1990) 82: 209–216.

Belch, J. J. F., D. Ansell, R. Madhok, A. O'Dowd, and R. D. Sturock. "Effects of altering dietary essential fatty acids with prostaglandin E_1 precursors cis-linolenic acid and gamma linolenic acid." *Scandinavian Journal of Rheumatology* (1988) 12: 85–89.

———. "Effects of altering dietary essential fatty acids on requirements for non-steroidal anti-inflammatory drugs in patients with rheumatoid arthritis." *Annual Rheumatology Disease* (1988) 47: 96–104.

Bittiner, B. S., I. Cartwright, W. F. G. Tucker, and S. S. Bleehen. "A double-blind, randomized, placebo-controlled trial of fish oil in psoriasis." *Lancet* (1988) 1: 378–380.

Bjorneboe, A., E. Soyland, G. E. A. Bjorneboe, G. Rajha, and G. Drevon. "Effect of dietary supplementation with eicosapentaenoic acid in treatment of atopic dermatitis." *British Journal of Dermatology* (1987) 117: 463–469.

Blackburn, M. "Uses of Efamol for depression and hyperactivity in children," in *Omega 6 Essential Fatty Acids*, edited by D. F. Horrobin. New York: Wiley-Liss, 1990, pp. 345–350.

Brush, M. G., Watson, D. F. Horrobin, and M. S. Manku. "Abnormal essential fatty acid levels in plasma of women with premenstrual syndrome." *American Journal of Obstetrics and Gynecology* (1984) 150: 363–366.

Cerin, A., A. Collins, B. M. Landgren, and P. Eneroth. "Hormonal and biochemical profiles of premenstrual syndrome: Treatment with essential fatty acids." *Acta Obstetrics and Gynecology Scandinavia* (1993) 72: 337–343.

Cupps, T. R., and A. S. Fauci. "Corticosteroid-mediated immunoregulation in man." *Immunology Review* (1982) 65: 133–155.

Dupont, E., L. Schandene, R. Devos, M. Lambermont, and J. Wybran. "Depletion of lymphocytes with membrane markers of helper phenotype: A feature of acute and chronic drug-induced immunosuppression." *Clinical Experimental Immunology* (1983) 51: 345–350.

Earle, C. M., E. J. Keogh, Z. S. Wisniewski, A. G. S. Tulloch, D. J. Lord, G. R. Watters, and C. Ghatthaar. "Prostaglandin E_1 therapy for impotence, comparison with papaverine." *Journal of Urology* (1990) 143: 57–59.

Fauci, A. S., and D. C. Dale. "The effect of in vivo hydrocortisone on subpopulation of human lymphocytes." *Journal of Clinical Investigation* (1974) 53: 240–246.

French, J. M. "MaxEPA in multiple sclerosis." *British Journal of Clinical Medicine* (1984) 38: 117–121.

Giron, D. J. "Inhibition of viral replication in cell cultures treated with prostaglandin E_1." *Proceedings of the Society for Experimental Biology Medicine* (1982) 170: 25–28.

Glen, E. M. T., L. E. F. MacDonald, A. I. M. Glen, and J. MacKenszie. "Possible pharmacological approaches to the prevention and treatment of alcohol-related CNS impairment," in *Pharmacological Treatments for Alcoholism*, edited by G. Edwards and J. Littleton. London: Croom Helms, 1984, pp. 311–350.

Godschalk, M., J. Chen, P. G. Katz, and T. Mulligan. "Prostaglandin E_1 as treatment for erectile failure in elderly men." *Journal of the American Geriatric Society* (1994) 42: 1263–1265.

Haynes, B. F., and A. S. Fauci. "The differential effects of in vivo hydrocortisone on kinetics of subpopulations of human peripheral blood thymus-derived lymphocytes." *Journal of Clinical Investigation* (1978) 61: 703–707.

Hedquist, P. "Effects of prostaglandins on autonomic neurotransmission," in *Physiological, Pharmacological and Pathological Aspects*, edited by S. S. M. Karin. Lancaster, England: MLTP Press, 1976, pp. 37–62.

Horrobin, D. F., L. G. Durand, and M. S. Manku. "Prostaglandin E_1 modifies nerve conduction and interferes with local anaesthetic action." *Prostaglandins* (1977) 14: 103–112.

Horton, E. W. "Actions of Prostaglandin E_1, E_2, and E_3 on central nervous system." *British Journal of Pharmacology* (1964) 22: 189–192.

Kremer, J. M., W. Jubiz, A. Michaslek, R. I. Rynes, L. E. Bartholomew, J. Bigavo, M. Timchalk, D. Beeler, and L. Linnger. "Fish-oil supplementation in active rheumatoid arthritis." *Annual Internal Medicine* (1987) 106: 497–503.

Kremer, J. M., A. V. Michalek, L. Lininger, C. Huyck, J. Bigauoette, M. A. Timchalk, R. I. Rynes, J. Zieminshi, and L. E. Bartholomew. "Effects of manipulation of dietary fatty acids on clinical manifestation of rheumatoid arthritis." *Lancet* (1985) 1: 184–187.

Kunkel, S. L., J. C. Fantone, P. A. Ward, and R. B. Zurier. "Modulation of inflammatory reaction by prostaglandins." *Progressive Lipid Research* (1982) 20: 633–640.

Kunkel, S. L., S. B. Thrall, R. G. Kunkel, J. R. McCormick, P. A. Ward, and R. B. Zurier, "Suppression of immune complex vasculitis in rats by prostaglandin." *Journal of Clinical Investigation* (1979) 64: 1525–1529.

Kuno, S., R. Ueno, O. Hayaishi, H. Nakashima, S. Harada, and N. Yamamoto. "Prostaglandin E_2, a seminal constituent, facilitates the replication of acquired immune deficiency syndrome virus in vitro." *Proceedings of National Academy of Science USA.* (1986) 83: 3487–3490.

Lee, T. H., R. L. Hoover, J. D. Williams, R. I. Sperling, J. Ravalese, B. W. Spur, D. R. Robinson, E. J. Corey, R. A. Lewis, and K. F. Austen. "Effect of dietary enrichment with eicosapentaenoic acid and docasahexaenoic acid on in vitro neurophil and monocyte leukotriene generation and neurophil function." *New England Journal of Medicine* (1985) 312: 1217–1224.

Manku, M. S., M. Oka, and D. F. Horrobin. "Differential regulation of the formation of prostaglandins and related substances from arachidonic acid and dihomo gamma linolenic acid: effects of ethanol." *Prostaglandins in Medicine* (1979) 3: 119–128.

Margaro, M., L. Altomonte, A. Zoli, L. Mirone, D. DeSole, G. Di-

Mario, S. Lippa, and A. Oradei. "Influence of diet with different lipid composition on neutrophil chemiluminescence and disease activity in patients with rheumatoid arthritis." *Annual Rheumatology Disease* (1988) 47: 793–796.

Nervi, A. M., R. O. Peluffo, and R. R. Brenner. "Effect of ethanol administration in fatty desaturation." *Lipids* (1980) 15: 263–268.

Neu, I. J. Mallinger, A. Wildfeuer, and L. Mehler. "Leukotrienes in cerebrospinal fluid of multiple sclerosis patients." *Acta Neurology Scandinavia* (1992) 86: 586–587.

Ochermann, P. A., I. Bachrock, S. Glans, and S. Rassner. "Evening primrose oil as a treatment of the premenstrual syndrome." *Rec. Advanced Clinical Nutrition* (1986) 2: 404–405.

Pluda, J. M., R. Yarchoan, E. S. Jaffe, I. M. Feuerstein, D. Solomon, S. M. Steinber, K. M. Wyvill, A. Raubitschi, D. Katz, and S. Broder. "Development of non-hodgkin lymphoma in a cohort of patients with severe human immunodeficiency virus (HIV) infection on long-term antiretroviral therapy." *Annual Internal Medicine* (1990) 113: 276–282.

Prickett, J. D., D. R. Robinson, and A. D. Steinberg. "Dietary enrichment with polyunsaturated acid, eicosapentaenoic acid prevents proteinuria and prolongs survival in NZBxNZW F_1 mice." *Journal of Clinical Investigation* (1981) 68: 556–559.

Pulse, T. L., and E. Uhlig. "A significant improvement in a clinical pilot study utilizing nutritional supplements, essential fatty acids, and stabilized aloe vera juice in 29 HIV seropositive ARC and AIDS patients." *Journal of Advanced Medicine* (1990) 3: 209–230.

Puolakka, J., L. Makarainen, L. Viinikka, and O. Ylikorkala. "Biochemical and clinical effects of treating the premenstrual syndrome with prostaglandin synthesis precursors." *Journal of Reproductive Medicine* (1985) 30: 149–153.

Rotrosen, J., D. Mandio, D. Segarnick, L. J. Traficante, and S. Gershon. "Ethanol and prostaglandin E_1: Biochemical and behavioral interactions." *Life Science* (1980) 26: 1867–1876.

Schroeder, H. C. "Avarol restores the altered prostaglandin and leukotriene metabolism in monocytes infected with HIV Type I." *Virus Research* (1991) 21: 213–223.

Segarnick, D. J., H. Ryer, and J. Rotrosen. "Precursor and pool-dependent differential effects of ethanol on human platelets prostanoid synthesis." *Biochemistry and Pharmacology* (1985) 34: 1343–1346.

Swank, R. L. "Effect of low saturated fat diet in early and late cases of multiple sclerosis." *Lancet* (1990) 336: 37–39.

Uda, R., S. Horiguchi, S. Ito, M. Hyodo, and O. Hayaishi. "Nociceptive effects induced by intrathecal administration of prostaglandin D_2, E_2, and F_2 alpha in conscious mice." *Brain Research Journal* (1990) 10: 26–32.

Volberding, P. A., S. W. Lagakos, J. M. Grimes, D. S. Stein, H. H. Balfour, R. C. Reichman, J. A. Bartlett, M. S. Hirsch, A. P. Phair, R. T. Mitsuyasu, M. A. Fischi, and R. Soeiro. "The duration of zidovudine benefit in persons with asymptomatic HIV infection." *Journal of the American Medical Association* (1994) 272: 437–442.

Williams, L. L., D. M. Doody, and L. A. Horrocks. "Serum fatty acid proportions are altered during the year following acute Epstein-Barr virus infection." *Lipids* (1988) 23: 981–988.

Wright, S., and J. L. Burton. "Oral evening primrose seed oil improves atopic eczema." *Lancet* (1982) 2: 1120–1122.

Ziboh, V. A., K. A. Cohen, C. M. Ellis, C. Miller, R. A. Hamilton, K. Kragballe, C. R. Hydrich, and J. J. Voorhees. "Effects of dietary supplementation of fish oil on neutrophil and epidermal fatty acids." *Archives Dermatology* (1986) 122: 1277–1282.

Ziboh, V. A. and C. C. Miller. "Essential fatty acids and polyunsaturated fatty acids: significance in cutaneous biology." *Annual Review Nutrition* (1990) 10: 433–450.

Zurier, R. B. "Prostaglandins, immune responses and murine lupus." *Arthritic Rheumatology* (1982) 25: 804–809.

———. "Eicosanoids and inflammation," in *Prostaglandins in Clinical Practice*, edited by M. B. Peterson, W. D. Watkins, and J. R. Fletcher. New York: Raven Press, 1989, pp. 79–96.

CHAPTER 16: THE ZONE AND LIFE EXTENSION

Books
Hayflick, L. *How and Why We Age.* New York: Ballantine, 1994.
Walford, R. L. *The 120 Year Diet.* New York: Simon and Schuster, 1986.
Weindruch, R., and R. L. Walford. *The Retardation of Aging and Disease by Dietary Restriction.* Springfield, IL: C. C. Thomas, 1988.

Articles
Cerami, A. "Hypothesis: Glucose as a mediator of aging." *Journal of the American Geriatric Society* (1985) 33: 626–634.
Kagawa, Y. "Impact of westernization on the nutrition of Japanese: Changes in physique, cancer, longevity, and centenarians." *Preventive Medicine* (1978) 7: 205–217.
Kemnitz, J. W., R. Weindruch, E. B. Roecher, K. Crawford, P. L. Kaufman, and W. B. Ershler. "Dietary restriction of adult male rhesus monkeys: Design, methodology and preliminary findings for the first year of study." *Journal of Gerontology* (1993) 48: B17–B26.
Laganiere, S., and B. P. Yu. "Anti-lipoperoxidation of food restriction." *Biochemistry and Biophysics Research Communication* (1987) 45: 1185–1189.
Langaniere, S., B. P. Yu, and E. J. Masoro. "Inhibition of membrane lipoperoxidation and modulation of antioxidant status by food restriction." *Fed. Proc.* (1987) 46: 567–570.
Lok, E., F. W. Scott, R. Mongeau, E. A. Nera, S. Malcolm, and D. B. Clayson. "Calorie restriction and cellular proliferation in various tissues of the female Swiss Webster mouse." *Cancer Letters* (1990) 51: 67–73.
MaCay, C. M., M. F. Crowell, and L. A. Maynard. "The effect of retarded growth upon the length of the life span and upon ultimate body size." *Journal of Nutrition* (1935) 10: 63–79.
Masoro, E. J., R. J. M. McCarter, M. S. Katz, and C. A. McMahan. "Dietary restriction alters characteristics of glucose fuel use."

Journal of Gerontology and Biological Science (1992) 47: B202–B208.

Masoro, E. J. "Food restriction and the aging process." *Journal of the American Geriatric Society* (1984) 32: 296–300.

Masoro, E. J., M. S. Katz, and C. A. McMahan. "Evidence for the glycation hypothesis of aging from the food-restricted rodent model." *Journal of Gerontology and Biological Science* (1989) 41: B20–B22.

———. "Retardation of aging processes by food restriction." *American Journal of Clinical Nutrition* (1992) 55: 1250S–1252S.

Reaven, E. P., D. Wright, C. E. Mondon, H. Ho, and G. M. Reaven. "Effect of age and diet on insulin secretion and insulin action in the rat." *Diabetes* (1983) 32: 175–180.

Reaven, G. M., and E. P. Reaven. "Prevention of age-related hypertriglyceridemia by caloric restriction and exercise training in the rat." *Metabolism* (1981) 30: 982–986.

Vallego, E. A. "La dieta del hambre a dias alternos en la alimentacion de los viejos." *Review of Clinical Experience* (1957) 63: 25–31.

Walford, R. L., S. B. Harris, and M. W. Gunion. "The calorically restricted low-fat, nutrient-dense diet in Biosphere 2 significantly lowers blood glucose, total leukocyte count, cholesterol and blood pressure in humans." *Proceedings of National Academy of Science USA* (1992) 89: 11533–11537.

Young, J. B., D. Mullen, and L. Landsberg. "Caloric restriction lowers blood pressure in the spontaneously hypertensive rat." *Metabolism* (1978) 27: 1711–1714.

INDEX